Special Praise for *Making Peace with Your Plate*

"*Making Peace with Your Plate* is a refreshing and meaningful book to help you or a loved one recover from an eating disorder. What makes this book stand out is its unique format of alternating chapters. There is a 'story chapter,' which chronicles Robyn Cruze's recovery, followed by a 'therapist chapter,' which offers practical tools from seasoned eating-disorder therapist, Espra Andrus. Together this unique approach creates a powerful synergy."

Evelyn Tribole, MS, RD
Coauthor of *Intuitive Eating*

"*Making Peace with Your Plate* is a refreshingly unique addition to the recovery bookshelf. Robyn and Espra not only provide much hope, but also concrete tools to help make recovery from eating disorders a reality."

Jenni Schaefer
Author of *Almost Anorexic, Life without Ed*, and *Goodbye Ed, Hello Me*

"I love how clearly this book explains recovery. When I was in treatment, I always asked 'What *is* recovery?' and nobody could answer that in the eating disorder world. This book will help you define recovery and give you tools for change."

Ashley Hamilton

"Read this book. It describes the war that rages inside individuals with eating disorders and common sense therapeutic approaches to intervene in that war. I recommend this book to anyone struggling with internal/interpersonal conflicts—regardless of their source."

Kay L. Dea, DSW
Professor and Dean Emeritus
University of Utah
College of Social Work

"This intriguing new book provides two parallel perspectives on recovery from an eating disorder. At times poetic but consistently grounded in the cutting edge of science and research, *Making Peace with Your Plate* is a richly human description of how eating disorders can affect the thoughts and feelings at the center of a sufferer's sense of self. It is especially helpful in that these profoundly personal reflections are matched with advice about practical skills for managing the challenge of full recovery."

Douglas W. Bunnell, PhD, FAED, CEDS
Chief Clinical Officer
Monte Nido & Affiliates

"*Making Peace with Your Plate* provides a unique and meaningful vantage point. You will feel understood as you read Robyn's account of her struggle with an eating disorder, and you will find practical tools in the chapters authored by Espra, an experienced eating-disorder therapist."

Jennifer L. Taitz, PsyD
Author of *End Emotional Eating: Using Dialectical Behavior Therapy Skills to Cope with Difficult Emotions and Develop a Healthy Relationship to Food*

MAKING PEACE
with Your Plate

MAKING PEACE
with Your Plate
EATING DISORDER RECOVERY

ROBYN CRUZE

and

ESPRA ANDRUS

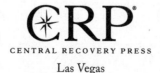

CENTRAL RECOVERY PRESS

Las Vegas

Central Recovery Press (CRP) is committed to publishing exceptional materials addressing addiction treatment, recovery, and behavioral healthcare topics, including original and quality books, audio/visual communications, and web-based new media. Through a diverse selection of titles, we seek to contribute a broad range of unique resources for professionals, recovering individuals and their families, and the general public.

For more information, visit www.centralrecoverypress.com.

Publisher: Central Recovery Press
           3321 N. Buffalo Drive
           Las Vegas, NV 89129

18 17 16 15   2 3 4 5

ISBN: 978-1-937612-45-0 (paper)
      978-1-937612-46-7 (e-book)

Photo of Robyn Cruze © Jim Paussa. Used with permission.
Photo of Espra Andrus © Nick Adams. Used with permission.

Publisher's Note: This book contains general information about addiction and other self-destructive behaviors, and developing wellness and emotional health. The information is not medical advice, and should not be treated as such. Central Recovery Press makes no representations or warranties in relation to any medical information in this book; this book is not an alternative to medical advice from your doctor or other professional healthcare provider.

If you have any specific questions about any medical matter you should consult your doctor or other professional healthcare provider. If you think you or someone close to you may be suffering from any medical or mental health condition, you should seek immediate medical attention. You should never delay seeking medical advice, disregard medical advice, or discontinue medical treatment because of information in this or any book.

Our books represent the experiences and opinions of their authors only. Every effort has been made to ensure that events, institutions, and statistics presented in our books as facts are accurate and up-to-date. To protect their privacy, some of the names of people, places, and institutions have been changed.

Cover design and interior by Deb Tremper, Six Penny Graphics.

Love to our devoted families, who urge and support us to
have the courage to follow our dreams and share our truth.

We lovingly commit this work to all individuals everywhere
who suffer with eating disorders, and to all those who
have been tricked into believing the lie that their worth
is defined by the size and shape of their body.

Table of Contents

Foreword

Robyn Cruze and Espra Andrus are wonderful women with much to share. Espra has been a trusted colleague and friend for about twenty-five years. When Espra first came to work with me and the staff at our eating disorder treatment center, I anticipated that we would be teaching her. Very quickly I learned that she would be the one doing most of the teaching. She is an astute and wise professional with a compassionate heart. I have more recently become aware of Robyn through her remarkable story. In this book she shares pieces of the puzzle of her life, which will have meaning in the lives of others whose stories also need to be embraced and told. Her story, and her storytelling, is compelling, touching, and impactful. The commentary provided by Espra completes each chapter beautifully.

These two powerful women have teamed up to bring us a rare and substantial work. *Making Peace with Your Plate* gives a breadth of knowledge and practical help for the illnesses of disordered eating, but it is also an inspiring story of the resiliency of the human soul. It provides evidence that an individual with tenacity and a willingness to be real can overcome human weakness, adversity, and pain and suffering; find peace and joy in his or her own life; and then extend that gift to others.

The authors take the reader on a journey into the severity, depth, and darkness of the eating-disorder illness. They help us understand its stark reality, its deadly nature, and its complicated maze of lies. They show us how to care for our bodies and minds, how to manage our emotions, and how to nurture relationships with self and others. They teach the skills and tools of recovery that can be applied in daily life. These principles and practices are the stepping stones out of these illnesses and into the hope and actuality of recovery. The reader will understand why it is important to take recovery steps, what steps can be taken, and how those steps can be taken.

This book may initially attract those whose lives have been touched by disordered eating. It will also be meaningful to those who have been touched by the suffering that comes with any addictive or mental illness. And it will be of great value to medical, dietary, and psychotherapy professionals. Within its pages are many nuggets of clinical wisdom that will help both novices and veterans in the healing arts.

Since I was a young boy, I have had a deep desire to sit at the feet of those individuals who seemed to have great wisdom. It started with listening to warnings and counsel from good parents. It continued with listening to stories told by grandparents who truly cared. Later, it included feeling connected to a teacher at school who went out of his way to reach out and help a struggling young teenager. Those connections meant the world to me. This deep desire continued through my college studies of religion, philosophy, psychology, and the effects of one's spiritual beliefs in the process of healing and creating a life of quality, fulfillment, and serenity. In this lovely book, I have once again been exposed to a sizable serving of practical wisdom. I commend these two resilient, brilliant, and kindhearted women for their significant contribution to our field.

Michael E. Berrett, PhD
Psychologist, CEO, Cofounder, Center for Change
Coauthor, *Spiritual Approaches in the Treatment
of Women with Eating Disorders*

Acknowledgments

We are so grateful for all the support and help of so many who made this book a reality. A special thanks goes to our families: Brenda, Tim, Lilly, and Chloe—we love you.

To the finest support team ever, David Nelson, Valerie Killeen, Lori Strawn, Michael Berrett, Melanee Cherry, and Hayley Giles; we are truly grateful for your expertise and your shared passion and encouragement in getting this book into the hands of those who need it most. It would have been impossible without the hours of consultation, review, and assistance you contributed. Thanks to the countless other professionals who have contributed their ideas and wisdom.

Robyn would like to give additional thanks: To my loving family for allowing me to bring you on this journey of sharing my story as I see it, and in turn yours. To my warrior sisters who have supported me within this journey of finding my voice, and encouraging me to share it: Andi (my other pea in the pod of life), Nicole Owenga-Scott, Emily Dykes, Roxane Wilson, Zoe Tryon, Stephanie Chao, and Nicole Rigato. I am indebted to all of you for your friendship, love, and personal wisdom. I love you. And to Lori and Earl Hightower: thank you.

Espra would like to give additional thanks: To Mom and Pop for your unwavering wisdom, confidence, nurturing, and support including during meltdowns. I am blessed to have you, and I love you to infinity. To my family and friends for enduring endless conversations about this work, your reassurance that my voice can make a difference, and for being the huge part of my fountain of blessings that you are. Thank you to the founders of Center for Change, my DBT consultation team, and the many clients, families, teachers, and colleagues who have trusted, believed in me, and passed on their wisdom and knowledge.

And to Francyne Cruze, who epitomized all mothers around the world who walk the path with their children in a desperate search in understanding and ending eating disorders. God bless you.

Introduction

Robyn

I gave my soul to my eating disorder. I truly believed I would die from my illness, as many do. I felt my heart being tarnished by the dictates of it, and I was sinking, along with all the dreams and purpose I once had. I was treading in the deep end of life with only my nostrils above the waterline. Like a caterpillar that never came out of its cocoon, I was lost in the darkness of isolation, never to become the butterfly that God intended me to be. That is, until recovery.

"*You* are the big, fat liar!" I declared holding my fork in mid-air victory. "I *will* eat this chicken. I will not purge, starve, binge, or—#@*! you—harm myself anymore!" Stabbing the chicken with conviction, I began to chew with a half-smile/half-snarl that left my illness speechless . . . . And just like that, without any massive event, my recovery began ten years ago. Here's the thing: I had attempted recovery many times before then, but only when I finally became willing to own my journey and felt a deep desire to reclaim myself did I begin to take back my life. I have not binged, purged, nor starved myself since.

Now having reached the other side of my recovery, I am humbled by the fact that there remains a cold, hard truth: Many of my sisters and brothers are still dying from eating disorders. The illness is still having its say, leaving many stuck in the illusion of control, false reality, and unrealistically high expectations of themselves and others. If only they could get into recovery and free themselves from the obsession of an eating disorder, life (with all its wonder and challenges) would be like reaching the end of the rainbow—a pot of gold, rich with their true selves, just waiting for them. But how do we get into recovery and stay there? How can I help others to stop suffering earlier on? How can I help break them out of the spell of their eating disorders?

I've found that there is no single, tangible method of recovering from eating disorders that covers all the stages of discovery required to find ourselves. But I also realize that many concepts for recovery are vital, even if they alone are unable to take us to the other side, where full recovery resides. To fully realize myself in recovery, I understood that the process needed to be adapted to my safety requirements and self-discovery along the way. In other words, I needed a plan that changed along with me. I also knew that this process was of no real use unless I also worked with a specialist to deal with the underlying issues of pain, addiction, and trauma. It is the yin and yang of recovery. Today, my life feels like it's been upgraded from black-and-white TV to a colorful surround-sound system with high-definition. Yet it didn't always feel like that during my recovery. Recovering from an eating disorder is like shaking out a rug under which you have stored all your dust and dirt for years. When you shake the rug, the dust and dirt are blinding. It is gritty, and particles fly everywhere.

Even after I had achieved seven years free from the eating-disorder behaviors, I still needed to address my depression and my on and off use of alcohol to medicate it. I checked myself into rehab with the help of friends and my husband, Tim. During my stay at Cirque Lodge in Utah, a counselor suggested I see someone at the Center for Change for an evaluation because I had a history of eating disorders and a fierce hate for being weighed. They wanted to be certain this was not a continuing obstacle in my recovery process. It was there that I met Espra. I met with Espra for a total of two hours, but I remember thinking, "Here is a woman who has taught me more about eating disorders than I already knew." Let's face it; many of us who have struggled with eating disorders have studied so much about our illness that we could have a degree in nutrition and eating-disorder psychology—we are perfect researchers, perfect students, and perfect eating-disorder conformers. But Espra brought with her years of knowledge and experience in eating-disorder treatment, Dialectical Behavior Therapy (DBT), and a glorious sense of humor that could pierce through the most resistant character. I felt like I had nothing to hide in my two hours with Espra. I had long before stopped running from my eating disorder, but she understood, without a shadow of a doubt, that the crumbs of the illness that still niggled at me—although they had no control over me—were lies of outlandish proportion. And just like that, the crumbs were blown away. Meeting Espra was a godsend, and without her this book would not be possible.

Despite the obstacles that come along with being human, I have made it through to full recovery. For me, *full recovery* means that my daily activities are no longer dictated by my body or food intake. It means that as a woman in today's society, I am still susceptible to the media and my peers' judgments, but they no longer define me. It means that my true self, not the words of the eating disorder, prevails. No one told me that full recovery was possible. No one told me that to be in recovery doesn't mean accepting yourself from the very beginning. That, in fact, is not possible. But to "own" your story is. No one told me that full recovery is a combination lock that, if I have the courage to open it, will allow the cocoon to slowly break and set me—a beautiful butterfly in my own right, with all my faults, passions, and uniqueness—free from eating disorders, ready to fly. This book is for you because I want you to know this. I want you to grab onto this information and breathe it in whenever you are in doubt or fear about the recovery process. I want you to know that you are worth recovery. That I believe in you. Believe it or not, the gifts are there, below the surface, waiting for you to own.

Espra

For years, the universe nudged me toward adding the treatment of individuals suffering with eating disorders to the focus of my work as a therapist. I resisted. Then life, with the tapestry it weaves from beauty and tragedy, outright catapulted me toward eating-disorder work. As a believer that we all have choices, I felt that I had two choices: 1) work with eating disorders or 2) work with eating disorders. As a recovering perfectionist, I chose both.

Almost two decades ago I sat at a boardroom table with the founders of Center for Change, a premier eating disorder treatment program in Utah. The founders, whom I admired both as clinicians and as people, had more than eighty years of collective clinical experience. As I confessed my inadequacies in treating eating disorders, one of them clarified, "If you weren't a good therapist, we wouldn't be having this conversation. We'll teach you what you need to know about eating disorders." And teach me they did; their wisdom and interventions often flowed out of them as casually as if they were telling me how to water a plant. Wishing my brain were a sponge, I watched my mentors as they worked, and I scribbled down their words. They watched over me, taught me, and tirelessly passed on their knowledge, mostly to quell my episodes of panic.

I have read and listened to the voices of internationally respected practitioners, researchers, and teachers in the field of eating-disorder treatment. I value staying apprised of developments in treatment and putting them into action. To improve my therapy skills, I completed intensive training in Dialectical Behavioral Therapy (DBT).

DBT has been shown to be effective in treating Bulimia Nervosa and Binge Eating Disorder. Although research has yet to solidify a therapeutic approach that shows overwhelming superiority in treating Anorexia Nervosa, many of my clients have appreciated the concrete nature of many of the DBT skills in their fight against their eating disorders.

My interventions come from traditional therapeutic modalities. Some tools were born in moments of inspiration or desperation, while in the trenches alongside clients, families, and colleagues on the eating-disorder battlefield. Many of the techniques I use I have learned from the most informed eating-disorder experts of all—my clients. Some of these experts have taught me in subtle and almost imperceptible ways, and others have taught me with passionate critiques.

Despite more than twenty years of training and practice, I don't feel like an expert in treating eating disorders. An expert, who had conquered her eating disorder after eighteen years of battling it, once entered my office. We spoke of her recovery journey, one that led her to a fulfilled life that had been free of eating-disorder behavior for seven years. We spoke of how lingering thoughts about her worth and value depending on her body size and shape—thoughts she knew to be untrue—grated on her nerves. She decided that I was an expert when I tossed a couple of ideas, which I'd seen as beneficial to others, her way. Robyn grabbed those ideas and ran with them.

One item on my list of sixty-seven things I want to do before I die is to write a book. So when Robyn's path again crossed with mine and she told me of her idea to write a book to help others recover from eating disorders, I thought the universe was urging me to pay attention.

Having fully recovered from her own eating disorder, Robyn felt that eating disorder recovery was an area of expertise for her, and she was right. Robyn wanted another voice to speak about recovery "from the other side of the therapist's couch," and wondered if I would consider being that voice. This was my dream, and it gave me permission to be imperfect, because Robyn was the expert. I knew I needed to accept the call.

Robyn and I share a passion: getting the message that it is possible to make a full and complete recovery from eating disorders into as many hands as possible. One way to do that is to expose the illusion and lies that eating disorders have sold to more than one out of every ten people, of all ages, in the United States.

I cannot begin to count how often I have clenched my teeth and snarled, like Robyn, "#@*! you, eating disorder, you're not going to win!" My hands throb, my eyes narrow, and my teeth are clenched even now as I catch myself pounding these words on my poor keyboard.

These amazing, intelligent, and talented people are victims of the eating disorder's lies—lies that convince them they are unlovable and worthless from the core of their being outward. The lie that if anyone catches on to who or what they really are, they will be quarantined, banned from love and acceptance, unless they can find a way to be good enough.

So often I have thought, *There's got to be something,* something *that I can do better or more intensely to shake the hearts of these beautiful souls. What can I do to help them see that eating disorders thrive on half-truths, lies, illusions, and discouragement? What can I do to help others step back and see a bigger picture that exposes the devastation (to ourselves, our loved ones, our children, and our society) that eating disorders leave in their wake? What can I do to help those who suffer with eating disorders see that full recovery exists, and that recovery has rewards that reach far beyond a mere existence of using sheer willpower to hold eating-disorder behaviors at bay?*

Recovery is more attainable to those who keep trying.

There is no formal definition of the exact point called eating disorder recovery, so both partial and full recovery are still defined based on an individual's experience of eating-disorder symptoms or the absence of symptoms. Not everyone recovers fully, but chances increase dramatically for those who enter the race, begin it, and stay in it. Recovery is more attainable to those who keep trying. Decrease eating-disorder behaviors, no matter how long it takes. Be willing to set goals to increase self-worth along the way. Neither Robyn nor I want to activate your shame and guilt and hopelessness by pretending that there are only two extremes in eating disorder recovery, full and complete recovery or failure. There are unlimited places in between that truly result in a better life.

In recovery you eat when you are physically hungry and stop eating when you are physically full, most of the time. You allow yourself to eat a wide range of foods rather than limiting yourself to a narrow range. When you eat more than your body needs, you do not punish yourself or compensate by ingesting more calories, spending calories, or restricting them later. You trust that it will sort itself out. Recovery means that you might be upset when you do not like the way your body looks or the way your clothing fits, but you get on with your planned activities instead of getting preoccupied with changing your body or eating differently. You engage in regular physical activity with the goal of enjoyment and life balance instead of spending calories. You are able to focus on your values, relationships, and priorities beyond the size or shape of your body regardless of your eating or how you feel about your body.

You can be in recovery or even fully recovered and still dislike parts of your body, want to be the best athlete, think about dieting, or sometimes use food to cope with emotions. The difference in recovery is that you are committed to recognizing the eating disorder's traps and doing whatever is necessary to steer clear of them or get out of them when you fall into them. Your energy, behaviors, and time revolve around your authentic values and priorities above making or keeping your body a certain way. For example, if I find a wallet with a hundred dollars in it my long-term values would lead me to return it, but I am certain the thought would occur to me that I could keep it. Once I observe the gap between my long-term values and my immediate thoughts and urges, I might call a friend and ask her to remind me that following my values, returning the money, would leave me feeling better in the long run. I might think I am bad or dishonest for having the thought to keep the money. Being who I want to be, however, is in what I do with those thoughts in my life. My clients generally agree that eating disorder recovery means avoiding eating-disorder behaviors even when thoughts or urges to do otherwise are present. Individuals generally consider themselves fully recovered when the thoughts and urges to engage in eating-disorder behaviors are merely a blip on the radar that uses no more energy than a fleeting irritation.

Both Robyn and I are convinced, and are committed to spreading the word, that there is hope in eating disorder recovery—not only hope of muddling through some miserable existence, but hope that there is a place for you in the world. Hope that you can feel that your life can have peace, fulfillment, and meaning without an eating disorder. I refuse to fall for the lie that eating disorders will prevail.

Anger gives us energy to push through obstacles that are in the way of our goals, and my anger, in part, has fueled this work. Both Robyn and I have channeled our anger to help us find courage, which is not necessarily a feeling. Courage, as any soldier fighting in a war will tell you, is not driven by emotion but by a decision made over and over to act. Some of my most courageous actions were taken when I was absolutely petrified! I believe that all people are born with blueprints, talents, and challenges from which to mold their destiny. I believe that if we can see them, tools are always available to help us, no matter what we have done before. I believe that we must be awake and act with courage as we see opportunities to align ourselves with our passions and values. It has taken courage for Robyn and me to embark on this journey of helping others find hope. And we invite you to come along with us.

Your world, your life, and your dreams
are right here waiting for you.

*Today I will allow myself to try something
different in order to claim my life.*

1.
Enough Already

Cory Jones and Hollywood Dreams

By Robyn

It all began outside the school canteen (cafeteria) as I sat bingeing on the five bags of potato chips that I'd purchased for recess. It was the first time I'd consciously decided to forgo my usual order of a sandwich for a larger quantity of food. The act was calculated and numbing. I was eleven years old.

As I remember it, Cory Jones was sitting across from me, trying to impress me by eating a fly. "Dare me to eat it?" he shot off. "Yeah," I muttered, in between shoveling in potato chips. I was in a comforting trance that I would later realize was telling of all my binges to come. Just a day or so prior, my mum had told our family that she might be dying from lupus (a potentially fatal autoimmune disease). There at the dining table, the night before Cory ate a fly, I was catapulted into a crippling battle with an eating disorder that I would fight until the age of twenty-nine.

Just like the definition of an alcoholic is different from that of a heavy drinker, so there is a difference between someone suffering from an eating disorder and someone who is preoccupied with his or her weight. In other words, I can be preoccupied with my food yet still understand and consider the consequences of my dieting and what it can do to my body and mind if I am not treating it correctly. If changes need to be made due to these consequences, although uncomfortable, I am able to make them for the better of my well-being. However, when I am eating disordered, I become dictated by the illness. I can weigh the costs and the benefits, but no matter what, the benefits of eating-disorder behavior appear to outweigh the costs.

For example: My friend Rebecca said to me one day, after I'd spent a Christmas holiday alone in a blackout from diet pills, "The difference between you and me, Robyn, is that I am not willing to kill myself to look good." I was. I didn't want to die, but I didn't care how close I came to death if it gave me a chance to be at the weight I believed I "should" be. This is the definition of an eating disorder in a nutshell.

My eating disorder took on many forms as I vacillated from binge eating to bulimia and, somewhere in there briefly, anorexia, or what I considered a "failed" anorexic. I chose what, to me, was the most powerful "f@#k it button," that which would place an immediate halt to my feelings. I chose what made me feel the most in control. It was that feeling of power that saved me from the reality that I actually had no control in my life—over my mum's health, my parents' rocky relationship, and most of all how people felt about me. Sometimes I felt like I had the eating disorder under control, that I could sustain the deprivation and grossly compromised living—and I found hope in it. Sometimes I let go of all control of food, life, and myself. I was not simply "conscious of my weight," I was living the life of the eating disorder, lost beneath the rubble of extreme illness and pain. Sometimes, too, I wanted to die because I saw no way out.

For the longest time, I wished I'd never had an eating disorder. I remember a day while working in Spain when I realized that my history was, well . . . mine. A history that I would never be able to change, no matter what I did. I was devastated about how my story looked and how my truth would sound to others. That in itself kept me fighting for control for more years than necessary. I didn't want to own my truth. I wanted someone else's story that looked more glamorous and successful than mine. I wanted to be like everyone in Hollywood, or at least the image I projected upon them.

I knew the manipulation that went along with modeling and the images in glamour magazines—the airbrushing that often took place after unimpressive photo shoots. I even knew this first-hand. I had been a professional TV and film actress. I knew the poses to strike during a photo shoot to make my jaw line look defined and pointy. I knew what angle the photographer needed to shoot to make me look rail-like. I knew that most of the "glamorous world" was smoke and mirrors; but somehow, I wanted to be the exception. I was seeking perfection, which would make me worthwhile. It was a state of mind that could never be obtained. The bar rose as my weight went down. It was all an illusion.

I believed that being thinner made me more lovable. Everyone said it wasn't the truth. I *knew* it was. I saw how my friends got more attention for being thinner and more beautiful. Or did I? Looking back, what I really saw were women who on the outside, appeared to be okay in their own skin, and that was stunning to me. I had never known what that felt like. These women didn't mope around, eye-balling others who looked at them. I wanted to know why everybody was looking at me. I wanted to know what they thought was wrong with me so I could change it and be everything to everyone. I got further and further away from reality because I was stuck in this tiny world of aiming to be someone who wasn't real. Do you see? I was stuck in a lie. I thought if I could just reach an ideal, then I could start living. But life was happening without me.

For many years I hid in the aphorism "tomorrow it will all be different." Life is difficult, and starting recovery is even more difficult. I know that to be true. But I also know that recovery is a place where you get to pardon yourself for not being perfect. Early recovery is like building faith in a power greater than yourself; you may catch glimpses of not feeling alone or miracles that touch you, but you cannot see this power of recovery, for it is not yet tangible, so it is a leap of faith. There will never be a "right" time to start recovery. I just had to make a decision, followed by an action and willingness to live life beyond food and body image and the intense pain from the shackles of the eating disorder. It takes hard work and commitment to be sure. But here's the thing: I was committed to my eating disorder for many years, and that was hard, too! The years I spent in the eating disorder were not worth it and never amounted to anything. Whether I was bingeing, purging, starving, or using alcohol and other drugs to prevent myself from eating, the outcome was the same. I got nothing, achieved nothing . . . except a story that I now get to change.

I spent many a day wondering, "Why?" Why did I get this eating disorder that made me dissociate from the world? Why, for such an intelligent person, did I become such an irrational mess when it came to what I looked like? I knew in my head the dysfunction of what I was thinking and doing, but my knowledge only got me a week or two of normality, at best, before going back to the insidiousness of it all.

I've wondered if it is because I have the addict gene pool in my family. Instead of primarily using alcohol or other drugs, my addict tendencies first appeared via obsession with food and then later my body size. Or maybe it was because when Mum, whom I depended on fervently, was diagnosed with lupus, I hardly cried. Instead, in disbelief that something so profoundly life-changing could happen, I coped with my overwhelming trauma and hushed the sheer panic by stepping into a cycle of binge-purge-starve. And though the fight for control provided me with a sense of achievement and control that was illusory, I was hooked. It's like the fact that I am not certain why my favorite color is green. Maybe it's because I was wearing green when I won the monkey bar race in second grade, and now I have formed a false belief that green is my favorite color. It's a story that hooked me, just as the lies of my eating disorder did.

So I can't spend my time on "why" anymore. Because spending more time on "why" takes valuable energy I no longer have the luxury or desire to give. That time and energy is what I need now, today, in this very moment to take me into the life that awaits me within my truth.

How to Follow Your Dreams and Not Your Critics

By Espra

Robyn's passionate story of her awakening and travels (wonderful and heartbreaking) along the path of her recovery is the foundation of this book. Robyn and I endeavor to create a way for you to see her path of struggle and recovery in action, as well as offer you tools to help you in your own recovery. We are both here to help you find your way, to encourage you and support you as you make your individual journey toward your own recovery.

The field of mental health is shifting to a view that learning and using skills and behaviors, rather than simply gaining insight, leads to behavioral and emotional change. So you see, this book is not about "why." It's about providing practical actions to help you pull away from the clutches of eating disorder. It is for helping you combine skills and willingness to do whatever it takes to put recovery first and go on to live your dreams.

Energy spent on repeatedly asking why you have an eating disorder, and waiting for the answer before you can start recovery, is energy misspent.

Velocity is dangerous without clear direction and a guide to get us where we want to go. You can put extreme effort into recovering from your eating disorder, but it may take you where you do not want to go. Thus your speed, energy, and hard work can work against, not in favor of, your recovery. As Robyn discovered, energy spent on repeatedly asking why you have an eating disorder, and waiting for the answer before you can start recovery, is energy misspent. Instead, taking small steps toward the destination you seek will keep you on target. Focus on questions such as, "What is the next action I need to take right now?" Persistently asking this question and finding even one small additional step to take in that direction is what recovery is made of.

If you are reading this book as someone who is suffering from an eating disorder, it is a great start. You are likely thinking in some way about recovery. Beginning to look at recovery starts with an event (external or internal) that you cannot afford to forget. For example, Robyn had a moment of awareness, a recognition of the chaotic insanity of the whole darn thing. This chaos is caused by the same eating disorder that promises to give you control over your life by managing your food, body size, or shape. There may be a sense of stepping back and seeing yourself lying, stealing, consuming, or avoiding food at any cost to your loved ones, relationships, or yourself. Perhaps you see that these are the very relationships, events, and opportunities that you desperately want to love and enjoy. Was there a catastrophe (related to your disorder) that occurred or that you barely avoided? Have loved ones told you how much your eating disorder is hurting them or that they are afraid for you? Did a significant other tell you that something has to give—the eating disorder or the relationship—or did a medical provider tell you that this really is a big deal because it is destroying your body? Regardless of the reason that brought you here, try not to judge whether your motivation is "right" or "wrong." (The eating disorder is probably already doing that for you!) The important thing is that you are here. Let's take it from this point.

We have included tools in each chapter that give you concrete ways to look at various parts of your eating disorder. With each tool, we ask you to look at your eating disorder as it affects you as a unique individual. Work with the tools in your own way, and keep them in one place as your tool kit for future use. You will need them throughout your recovery. Here is your first tool:

 Think about the events or thoughts that made you consider recovery. There is no right or wrong answer. What occurred the instant before you said, "Enough! That's it!"? Write it down. Then write it on several sticky notes or cards. Put them on your mirror, in your wallet, in your car, or wherever you look throughout the day. Begin to bombard yourself with this information until it becomes your automatic thinking.

Do everything possible to read and remember your motivation and be prepared. You cannot afford to forget what made you decide to take back your life.

• •

This tool will help you get what you need, just like Robyn who found what she needed—a way to sustain her decision. When the power of the moment passes, these reminders of the price you have paid for your eating disorder will be fuel that will help you find motivation again. A big part of recovery is finding ways to discover and fuel motivation when it sneaks out or runs away. If you don't, your eating disorder will smugly step back in without you noticing.

Each second brings a new chance to choose and to act in the direction of recovery, no matter what happened the moment before. Even the moments when you trip, fall, or stop to rest must not be confused with quitting the race. Recovering from this eating disorder takes a lifelong commitment, a day at a time, or sometimes, a second at a time. There is no single solution that covers all eating disorders, or all individuals. However, we believe that our guidelines, if used and committed to (again and again), will help you find and maintain long-term recovery. I predict that you will box yourself in at times by telling yourself that you are different, that your eating disorder is more harsh or more powerful—or not as harmful—and that you really are worthless and unlovable. Please believe me . . . *this is not the truth!* Right now, Robyn and I need you to trust us. And we promise, with time, you will begin to be able to trust yourself.

So, enough! No amount of controlling, restricting your food, or binge eating will remove your fears or make you a better person. It is draining and creates no lasting change. There is no solid ground to be found where your eating disorder will allow you to feel as if you have arrived at the place where you are enough. The scale will not define your worth or the amount of love you receive from other people. And eating disorders cannot be, never have been, and never will be cured by attempting to control your body or by being "better" at dieting. The idea that it is even possible is a lie, and you've been cheated. It's time to start this journey, one that really can help you take back your life. Your dreams are waiting. Robyn and I promise to show you ways to take what seems impossible and help it seem possible, and also doable, in a most liberating and inspiring way.

You are well on your journey now.

Doing something despite the fear of failure is success.

Today I will take on the very task I fear I cannot do. With this courage, I will write a new story for myself and my life, where anything can happen, where anything is possible . . . especially recovery.

2.

Take a Stand

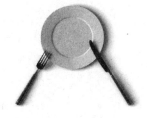

Jarred Marshmallow and Maltese Hips

By Robyn

It took many years for me to get to a place where I was ready to take the necessary steps toward recovery. Even when I felt I had had enough and could not go down the dark hole of despair any further, I was still waiting for a feeling of willingness. I wanted to experience a fight in me so powerful it would ignite something primal within, something that could make me resistant to the voice that told me I could not succeed. It was true that during the eighteen years of my eating disorder, I had moments of "success"—times my eating disorder celebrated, like when I reached a goal weight or, even better, below. These successes, however, were only big enough to keep me hooked to my illness, and far apart enough to fuel my obsession further—kind of like the rabbit chasing a carrot on a stick.

I was scared. I was petrified of how I would look if I allowed myself to honor what my body was telling me, my "body's mind." Hell, I didn't even know that my body had its own intelligence that could actually tell me what it needed to eat, if I listened. Even if this enlightening piece of physiological truth had penetrated my mind, I wouldn't have trusted it. I really believed I was different. *I mean, look at my gene pool*, I said to myself, *I am part Maltese. I am supposed to have large hips and round cheeks (on both ends)!* The truth is that genes will always influence our size. There is no way of changing bone structure. The insanity for me was that I was convinced that I had the ability to starve off my destiny of large hips and a lady mustache. In fact, I still had hips, even at my thinnest.

(Though I had never had a trace of facial hair—that was all in my head.)

An atmosphere of urgency began to permeate me. I had a deep need to get on with my life. I had wasted so much of my time. It created an anxiety in me that made me scramble for solutions in quick fixes. I imagined the time it would take to wade through the mess of my illness and seek recovery. This was time I didn't have the luxury of losing. It truly felt like recovery (the long way) would take truckloads of time and effort I did not have to give.

If I could just get to the ideal weight first, *then* I would be able to commit to recovery. *Seriously, how can I live with myself as I am and be okay?* I thought. Reaching my ideal weight would free me from the hourly obsession about how I looked, and the calculating and reviewing of food I ate or didn't eat. It would free me from the daydreaming about what I would achieve once I hit my perfect weight, how I would maintain my perfect weight once I got there (and I *would* get there this time), why it would all work out, what people would think of me then, what I would think of me then . . . *When I reach my perfect weight, I will be free and ready to move forward.* It made perfect sense to me. This became my every breathing moment's goal. But little did I know I would never, ever achieve it. It was like trying to catch a genie to grant me wishes—they aren't real, so it was never possible.

And so spiraled my life. My isolated existence brought with it darkness brushed with tiny sparks of light that were just enough to keep me from ending it all. The highs usually came when I succeeded in starving myself for some precalculated, nonsensical period of time, or while I binged as I read the next new, hopeful fad-diet book. The new diet plan provided an elaborate and convincing explanation of why I couldn't lose weight any other way (and I feared that if I didn't have something that provided me hope and a solution straight after a binge, such as a new diet to start over with, I would not be able to endure the pain of sitting with the shame and hatred for myself that followed.) Then I would declare: "This time it will be different."

But I was always left in the same place. Nothing changed. I was convinced I was still a nobody, a failure, a reject. I would again be thrown into the dull madness of feeling lost at sea, deep in my illness. I embodied hopelessness, wearing it as if it were my life costume as I desperately struggled to gain the control that I'd never had. The time I was so passionate about saving was the very time I was wasting.

I floundered in that torturous sea for years, my head bobbing up and down, as glimpses of the shores of recovery teased me. It was so hard for me to understand the need to let go. Wouldn't I drown? That's how it felt.

Each time I binged, purged, or starved, the aftermath was the same. My skin would begin to crawl with a familiar, fierce sensation that made my heart pick up speed. I felt as if I were about to lose my mind. It made me want to spit on my own face and punch it unmercifully. But instead, I self-medicated and fed the beast. If I starved, I binged to medicate. If I binged, I purged to medicate. Sometimes I would just lie there bloated, conquered, ashamed, feeling outright insane and out of control—breathing erratically through the residue of anesthetized emotions that threatened to send me crazy forever. In my darkest moments, I would welcome it. Then, the cycle would begin again.

The cycle was the same every time; only the location differed. I would get angry. I would promise myself that I would never do it again. I'd get a day or two of "greatness," where starvation would act as false self-esteem. (One bite of food and it would be all over, of course.) I'd feel better. Then a feeling would come, and I would start emoting. I didn't like it. So once again, I'd act out via my trusted eating-disorder behavior. This cycle confirmed that I was saying yes to misery and possible death.

The mental anguish was taking its toll on me. I was beyond tired of a fight that felt unwinnable. For years my battle was about mastering my illness to ultimately gain control, happiness, and victory. Later it just became about surviving.

This new level of awareness that I was killing myself by choice now slept with me, and when I woke, I was fully conscious while making choices in my eating disorder. It was the same feeling as lying to a loved one's face during an argument. The feeling of being dishonest would stick to my being like unwashed vomit and its smell under my nails after a purge. I was shifting out of denial and into reality.

It was not a particularly special day when I declared defeat. The night before, I had binged on some jarred marshmallow from the dollar store and awoke covered in sweat. I had given myself food poisoning and was vomiting in a friend-of-a-friend's bathroom, someone who had graciously allowed me to stay in her home during my visit to Los Angeles. I had spent my last "dignity dime" on an illness that promised me the goods of perfection. There, at this generous stranger's home, I slid to the bathroom floor, robbed, knowing that without a doubt I had been scammed. Like anyone who has been robbed, I started to review how it could have happened to me.

In a moment of clarity, I understood that I had wanted what the eating disorder was selling. Unfortunately for me, the potion it sold was nothing but candy water disguised as a magic cure. I kept buying what the dodgy salesman in the cheap white suit was selling long after realizing that the goods were bogus. That was my part.

I was twenty-nine, severely depressed, broken, and clueless as to who I really was. I didn't have it in me to muster up that kick-ass fight I believed I needed to begin recovery. I was exhausted. After all, I had been fighting since I was eleven years old. I sat, breathless, in a moment of "oh so familiar." And then, I had a thought that I had never experienced: *What if I said no to my eating disorder? What if I could stop doing what it told me to do? If nothing else, I could do that.* Right there, having calmly stumbled upon my masked truth, a newfound hope blossomed. There was an unexpected shift in me. I had my hands on a simple action I could take. It was a key to my personal treasure. Like a hostage who has no more strength but has the ability to refuse to talk, I was now considering turning *against* my eating disorder and finding the power in saying no to it. I knew how my life looked when I was the "yes-man." I didn't want to do what my eating disorder asked of me anymore, so I said *NO.* The price, I realized, was way too high. Besides, I was bankrupt.

I so desperately wanted to experience life without the shackles of my eating disorder. I wanted to live, not just survive. The search for perfection was killing me, and honoring no one. I was trying to control something that I never had any power over. All my attempts were futile and full of consequences I could no longer face. There on the kind stranger's bathroom floor, I understood for the first time that I may not be able to control my eating disorder, but I could ignore it; I could walk away. I physically put my hands up with a sense of letting go. I didn't know how I would get to the happiness I longed for, but I realized that my eating disorder wouldn't be the way to get me there either. I had proof of that.

Put the Lid on the Jar of Marshmallows

By Espra

"Liar! You *%#@* liar! You lied to me!"

My stomach dropped, my breath caught in my chest, and I got chills as the core truth of the words hit me. My stomach dropped again when I realized that anyone within a city block must have wondered what lie I had told the woman in my office to bring out such rage.

My first interaction with Robyn involved an angry eruption so deep and heartfelt, the impact was like an explosion detonating behind my office door. Robyn was a self-taught expert on the complex and challenging issues of recovery. She was now on a soul-searching journey to find answers to lingering questions, and to still the nagging inner voice that had refused to shut off, even though Robyn had not engaged in eating-disorder behavior for seven years.

Robyn was forthright about what was on her mind. "I battled my eating disorder for more than a decade, and I have not engaged in eating-disorder behaviors for seven years. I no longer allow an eating disorder to run my life. I am in recovery," she stated proudly, with strength and gratitude. But Robyn also felt haunted. "I know without a doubt that my value and worth do not depend on my weight or size. But still, I have this niggling voice in the back of my mind that says they do. I know it makes no sense, but I am struggling to be rid of it." Unfortunately, this made perfect sense to me. These remnants so often cling to the minds of those in recovery, even in the latter stages.

Disgusted by eighteen years of lies from her eating disorder, Robyn knew not to believe them. "I want to tell the eating disorder to leave my head the hell alone," she said. That seemed like a brilliant idea to me, so I initiated an intervention often used in eating-disorder treatment:

I grabbed a chair, threw a pillow into it, and indicated that it now represented her eating disorder.

"Don't tell me. Tell the eating disorder," I challenged. "Say it with the exact words, intensity, and volume that match how you feel. Don't exaggerate, but don't hold back or filter your words. Don't worry about my naive ears; just tell it what you need to say."

Robyn didn't seem to worry at all about my naive ears as she suddenly clenched her fists and erupted, "Liar! You *%#@* liar! You lied to me!"

Robyn was livid. She was seeing the eating-disorder lies, and she was standing up to them. It was this anger that gave her the strength to set her roots more deeply into her recovery. It was standing face to face with the enemy within herself, the eating disorder, that helped her find the peace that could only be found in her own inner power—her authentic power. Anger can be scary, yet it is useful in that it gives you the energy to push through a barrier that stands in the way of accomplishing an important goal in your life. This energy is exactly what you will need if you are going to fight this eating disorder. You cannot meekly tell a powerful dragon that you want it to please leave you alone and expect that it will back off. I am not saying that you have to scream or curse in order to stand up to your eating disorder. Do it your own way; just be sure to stand up to it like you mean it.

If It Sounds Like an Eating Disorder, Chances Are It Is

Eating Disorder: "Lies, *lies*? These women are crazy. I'm the only one who tells you the truth. That's why you need me."

Truth: This statement is just one example of the way an eating disorder's lies can become exhausting mantras. The thoughts are yours (and not to be confused with "hearing voices" or having a separate personality), but they are so clear and powerful, it is like they are their own entity. That's why some people find it helpful to combat their eating-disorder thoughts as if they are a distinct or separate persona. Other people work with their eating disorder as if it is a part of their brain, with which other parts of their brain are caught in a tug of war. It is important for you to come to an understanding of the best way for you to conceptualize and work with your own screaming, whispering, internal eating-disorder voice. We will mostly refer to these patterns of thoughts as "the eating disorder." You will get scared as you examine your own eating-disorder lies in writing, notice the sheer number of them, and recognize their familiarity. Try hard not to let them scare you away from this journey. Your eating disorder has used these lies to keep you submissive to it, and it will use the same tricks to try to block your path to recovery.

If you struggle with an eating disorder, the following eating-disorder quotations will resonate with you in an eerily familiar way. If you do not suffer from an eating disorder yourself, they might make no sense at all. Use the quotations to try and touch the agony of having such brutal and unrelenting thoughts in your head.

In my professional journey, I've seen that eating-disorder thoughts rarely have more than a small strand of truth, around which a tapestry of deceit is woven. You cannot expect to see the lies until you start to pull away from the disorder's grasp and see the bigger picture. So let my examples of a typical eating-disorder voice guide you in becoming more conscious of your own.

Consider committing to doing something very different than what you've done in the past. Here's your chance to make a move. Open your mind. Be aware of your eating-disorder thoughts and question their accuracy. See if doubt enters your mind. You may just catch the eating disorder in one of its lies.

Recovery Does Not Equal Fat

Eating Disorder: "They are going to try to get you to gain weight, throw away everything you've worked so hard to create, and do that 'accept your body because you are wonderful on the inside' crap! Feeling okay about a fat, gross, and disgusting body will only make matters worse for you."

Truth: Recovery does not mean you will start eating, lose control, gain weight, and never stop. Nor does recovery guarantee that you will not need to go above whatever weight, size, or measurement your eating disorder has imposed on you. (I'd love to see the eating disorder's book of logic: How does it pick appropriate weight, size, measurement, or intake goals, anyway?) My clients frequently say they could recover if they knew for sure they wouldn't have to gain weight, or wouldn't gain and gain weight and never stop. I wish so badly there was a way to calm this terror before you walk headlong into it. Reassure yourself, if needed, by telling yourself that you are not stuck forever with anything that only brings you misery.

Recovery is about learning who you are and living a life that lines up with your long-term goals and values. You may notice thoughts that you need to get skinny "enough" before you start recovery, that you are too fat to have an eating disorder, or that you are too fat for others to believe you have one. These are eating-disorder thoughts, and they are backwards. The eating disorder makes it seem like being skinny enough is the solution that will make everything okay. You must find a way to step back from this belief and see that the eating disorder, not the size or shape of your body, is now the cause of your problems. It keeps you from seeing the actual problems. Perhaps it convinces you that if you could stop bingeing, have more discipline, or just eat less, you would no longer need to purge. (And for the record, just in case your eating disorder tells you that purging is only throwing up, purging is any behavior that you use to rid your body of unwanted calories. It can include laxatives, exercising, and numerous other behaviors.)

It is amazing that you will even consider recovery when you are terrified it will make you fat. Good for you! Both Robyn and I want to be clear that there is no guarantee that you will lose weight or that you won't need to gain weight, depending on your circumstances. Robyn and I do promise that our goal is not to get you to be okay with being "fat." I promise that I will teach you how to keep your eating disorder from calling the shots on what is or is not in your body's best interest. I guarantee that it is possible to learn how to give your body what it needs by eating when you are physically hungry and stopping when you are physically full, most of the time. When you do this, your body will settle into its balanced place. In that balanced place, your body will have the strength and stamina to do the things it needs and wants to do without running out of fuel and without hauling around fuel that it doesn't need. This is the best Robyn and I can give you, and we hope that it is enough to keep you moving toward recovery.

It Takes as Long as It Takes

Eating Disorder: "Your new job starts in three weeks. By then, if you work hard enough and do this right, you can crank through recovery, get this behind you, and be ready to start your new job and your new life."
Truth: I wish I could give you an estimated "time of arrival" for your recovery, but there truly is no time frame. It takes anywhere from months to years, and the most helpful mindset is that it takes as long as it takes, so stick with it. The reason is, each person has their own lock, and its combination is discovered along the journey. You have to find it, and you will, along the way. Recovery isn't a nice, clear picture of your identity, your passions, or your life's purpose that suddenly shows up one moment. These images start to form while you are busy trying to find them.

It is like having a box that has a picture of a completed puzzle on its front, while you only have a couple of pieces in your hand. You'll need to commit to searching for the other pieces. During your search, a time will come when you look around and see little shimmers of light starting to peek through, revealing parts of the picture that have been created by starting to put together the many pieces of you. Recovery is subtle. If you are working at recovery, please trust that positive changes are happening. You will begin to see glimpses of liberation and peace as you put more and more pieces together.

Take heart from the wisdom of my clients, who often reprimand me when I try to encourage them to use the "one day at a time," principle from twelve-step programs: "One day at a time? Hell, a day is an eternity! It's got to be one minute at a time, and sometimes even one second at a time!" They feel this approach respects the intensity of their personal fight. There's no right or wrong. Do whatever it takes for you to feel supported and encouraged . . . as long as you are not taking direction from your eating disorder. And if you need to take it one second at a time, then do it. *Just stay in the race.*

One way that urgency with time is important, though, is with making commitments and finding ways to stay motivated. Those things cannot wait. Do not sit and wait to feel motivation before you act. Instead, use action as a way to create and sustain motivation. Then, over time, your actions will **Action, more often** change your feelings in a "fake it till you make **than thinking,** it" kind of way. This approach works more **creates motivation.** quickly than trying to change your feelings by first changing your thoughts (although that strategy doesn't hurt, either). One of my colleagues explains this phenomenon by saying, "I am never more motivated to clean my kitchen than after I start to clean my kitchen."

We will continue to remind you that action, more often than thinking, creates motivation. Tough things are easier to put off until tomorrow, with the hope that we will feel stronger motivation by then. Before you know it, another year has passed.

The important thing to know is that people can and do make a full recovery from eating disorders. When you stay in the race, you are taking positive steps toward stopping eating-disorder behaviors in their tracks. You are then within recovery. It's that simple. And that difficult.

What commitment are you willing to make right now, regardless of the time involved? You may notice judgments that your commitment is too "dumb" or too "small" to consider. Your commitments must come from you alone, and not from what you think you "should" commit to, or what you think someone else wants. Unless you can make a commitment that is true for you, there will not be enough fuel to sustain you in your journey.

 Think about any commitments, large or small, you are willing to make. Write two of them on a card or in a journal and read them often. Believe me, you will surely need it.

Examples of commitments:
- Get rid of this eating disorder at any cost.
- Read my reasons to recover every day in order to build my willingness to recover.
- Commit to investigating who I am aside from the eating disorder, even though it's scary.
- Decrease bingeing, restricting, or purging.
- Reduce my self-punishment.

• •

Why Now?

Eating Disorder: "Just get these few pounds off, get this job, and get your career and your relationships on track. You will have what you need to be happy and won't need me after that."

Truth: Why recover now? So you do not lose one more moment of your life! Your eating disorder makes you and those around you miserable, and recovery may be the most difficult battle of your life. So enough! Let's look at the lies, expose the illness for what it truly is, and get you going toward uncovering "you."

Willpower is your attempt to control the eating disorder. It's helpful, but will only take you so far. You need more. So take a step back (even if you are trembling as you do so), take a stand against your eating disorder, and claim your power. The rest of your life is waiting.

My story may not show on my face.
It may not show in my voice.
But it always shows in my actions.

Right now, I have the opportunity to start my day in recovery with my best foot forward.
Right now, I choose to let go of the past and claim responsibility for my own actions.
I now own my life, my story, and my recovery.

3.

It's Not About the Food.
And It Is About the Food.

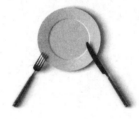

Sunny Days and an Unwanted Houseguest

By Robyn

My need to recover eventually became greater than my need to be thin. But I still had an overwhelming amount of fear that at times felt like an assailant sneaking up and choking me from behind, its grip squeezing the very life out of me. It was an intense fear motored by extreme anxiety. Some say it is healthy to have some fear and respect for an illness that can kill you. I had that. I respected that it went to any lengths to keep me within its clutches, and I feared that I would die a slow death—or worse, continue to live as I was—if I did not do something about it now.

My eating disorder was like a guest I'd invited to party at my home on weekends, but who ended up living there permanently, rent-free. Then slowly, quietly it began to dictate my every move. At the beginning of its stay, my guest was fun and promised me a good time and ways to feel like I fit in. I welcomed that. And then it turned on me when I didn't want to do the things it wanted me to do. Somehow we had become a team, and that team had an unbreakable code and an unspoken contract of free residency for the eating disorder at my expense. It was like the character in the movie *Single White Female*—nasty, coaxing, and possessing intent to kill. It said no one would like me because I was a fat, lazy loser. It said that I would never amount to anything because I couldn't control myself. It said that no one respects a person who can't look after herself and achieve such a simple task as a perfect weight. It said it was pointless for me to continue living, that I should kill myself and save my loved ones the misery of having to be so disappointed in me. But maybe, just maybe, I would get somewhere if I took its advice, because I knew nothing. I was nothing. I knew the eating disorder was right. It was, after all, just telling me what I already believed.

And like in other abusive relationships, I lived with the eating disorder knowing I would do anything it said in order to get and keep my goal weight, and attempt to earn self-esteem, respect, and love from others in the process. I needed to be liked because I was too fragile to handle indifference. My eating disorder promised me that I could be everything. I knew a few years into it that I would never be everything to everyone, but I kept trying. "This time it will work," it promised me. I knew it wouldn't, but I did it anyway. What else could I do? Sit with myself? Stand up for myself? I didn't have it in me. Besides, I knew I couldn't do it alone. Being thin felt like the only chance I had to start over and begin living my life. It was like buying tickets to win the lottery in order to be able to live in financial abundance, only buying the tickets was making me broke. I wound up broke and broken.

With all the fear and uncertainty I had, I also found a great amount of willingness and fight in me when I realized that my eating disorder was a liar. I held on to this, as I reminded myself that I would not die like this, and I would not live like this either. I secretly began to store any evidence of my abusive tenant's behavior that could be used in the court of human-dignity law. The eating disorder needed to be removed, but I had to be smart about it. I had tried before and it had failed. It always failed.

If I truly wanted to have recovery, I had to be willing to do something different.

Now I had to do something different. It was time to fight back, take back my home, the sacred temple that is called my body, and if that meant that I needed to eat food and sit (as scary as that felt) with it, I would. Because the truth is, whatever I fear is never as bad as I think it will be when I finally walk through it, and if I truly wanted to have recovery, I had to be willing to do something different.

I wanted so much to be able to eat normally. I wanted to start eating whatever I wanted, whenever I wanted, but I wasn't there yet. I had chosen to stop listening to the lies of the eating disorder, and now I had to stop lying to myself. I had long ago lost the connection with my body's signals. It had been screaming for years, and I chose to ignore it, so I knew that I would have to make myself safe first. Safety meant providing a structure that also allowed some freedom. It would keep me safe mentally, but also keep the eating disorder's voice quiet. Unbeknown to the eating disorder, I prepped for its eviction.

And then I did it. I forced the eating disorder out. I evicted the tenant by beginning to do the exact opposite of what it would have me do. I started eating three meals a day whether I wanted to or not. With every meal came a knock at the door from the eating disorder: it wanted to move back in. "You are a liar," I would state matter-of-factly, closing the door on it. It was like a vampire. It could not come in if I didn't invite it.

I started walking for forty-five to sixty minutes each day—any more would invite the eating disorder back home. I also stopped drinking alcohol because I had a tendency to replace one crutch with another. This desire to "switch the witch for the bitch" was always there. Just because I was making inroads to recovery didn't mean I didn't have a deep desire to numb my feelings. Drinking alcohol often took the place of my disordered eating in times when my food was "under control." It became the thing I used to numb myself so as not to feel my emotions. So I had to say no to that, too.

I had done so much research on what the media labeled "good" and "bad" diet foods that I could have taken nutritional exams and passed with flying colors. I had to place all the information that I had gathered during the years of chronic dieting aside and commit to starting from scratch. At first it was like trying to erase permanent marker from a white leather sofa. I had to attempt to erase all that I thought I knew and take small steps, steps that were not dictated by the eating disorder, as much as possible. The marker still faintly showed upon the white leather, but I had to trust that over time it would fade into nothingness.

I tried weighing and measuring my food and found that it triggered me. I tried mindful eating and found that I was ultimately starving myself because my body wasn't creating hunger signals yet. Deprivation meant depression, and my recovery meant not having to self-impose mental or physical pain any longer. When I finally embraced the concept of eating three meals a day, it provided me with a structured freedom that removed much of my shame and guilt. It allowed me, for the first time, to have a say in what I ate, yet also have the structure that I craved. I began to make peace with my plate.

During my stay in Los Angeles, I ended up living in the kind stranger's house for three months. Jessica was in her mid-thirties, exotic looking, with luscious black hair (the type you would see in a shampoo commercial). She was a unique, creative woman with a passion to nurture others. Her quirky sense of humor and forthrightness made me feel comfortable and safe. I knew where I stood with her, and I liked that. Jessica had become my dear friend and confidante when I needed it the most. It was summer in Los Angeles, a city where the temperature often reached the high nineties. Taking my daily walk with Jess, I could feel the weight of the world sliding off my shoulders and a sense of well-being in my body. I was happier, mostly free from the bondage of my illness, and in the moment. It was a rare feeling I had started to experience, walking around Silver Lake, with a delicious breeze kissing me in between my shoulder blades. In that moment, it felt symbolic for me to start getting more intimate with my own life. I felt like I didn't have a problem. But just as fast as I had that thought, it was replaced with a sudden urge to protect myself. I sensed danger. I had been here before. Just moments after feeling like I had achieved something, the eating disorder came lurking. Again I was reminded that I was on a journey of recovery, not yet at my destination.

Many teachers, gurus, and masters who have gone before us say that it is helpful to remember where you came from. I remembered all the pain and numbness, anxiety, depression, disgust, despair . . . along with momentary satisfaction from hitting the "right" number on the scale. I especially had a great sense memory for all those times I was in a relationship and "skinny." They were highlighted experiences that held a powerful sensation that I had "arrived." The feeling was something I equated to becoming a celebrity.

Nonetheless, I was now officially on my recovery journey. I was ready for my houseguest (now trespasser) to stay away. After all, here's what the eating disorder had offered me: Reaching my goal weight by eating only apples every day. (This ended in a binge.) Freedom to eat all I desired by purging everything back up. (This resulted in swollen face, scratched throat, bloating, bad breath, and a chronic starving sensation.) I had tried pretending that everything had cigarette ashes or burnt matches in it, because I hated anything to do with smoking, so that I would not want to eat it. I had tried looking in the mirror and telling myself how disgusting I was. Sometimes, I would even punch myself in the head. I tried things I never should have enacted upon my body, and I did things that amplified the disrespect and contempt I had for my body and myself. Ultimately, my illness had left me hopeless, locked in my bedroom alone, calling the suicide hotline; spending six hours at a time staring down at the toilet bowl; roaming dark city streets in search of a gas station so I could get food after a night out drinking. (I was defenseless and outright careless when I drank—not caring felt better than feeling.) Despite all that I knew about the eating disorder, when the rubber had hit the road and it was time to talk about food, I was petrified.

This time, however, I would not give up on myself.

This time, I would put my claws into recovery and hold on tight for dear life.

This time, I was willing to go to any lengths to get my life back.

How to Free Yourself from a Household Pest

By Espra

Right Now It Has to Be About the Food

Eating Disorder: "Sure this tastes good, but you don't deserve it. Well, eat it and enjoy it now that you've started. Just decide how you will make up for losing control."

Truth: Eating disorder recovery is not just about food, but it is impossible to recover when the eating disorder is choosing what, when, and how you eat.

During eating disorder recovery, total abstinence from food is clearly not an option. My clients get extremely frustrated that their eating disorder recovery requires healing their relationship with food, while at the same time having to be exposed to and continue to use the object of their addiction. Whether you battle urges to have more, less, or none at all—you still have to face food and you have to eat, no matter what.

We are talking about stabilizing your nutrition by eating a range of foods in adequate portions and on a regular schedule. Robyn realized the necessity of creating safety for her body by eating to

For your safety, it is essential for you to work with both a physician and a registered dietitian with specialized training and experience in treating eating disorders.

give her the mental, emotional, spiritual, and physical strength to fight her eating disorder. I strongly recommend that you also create your personal plan with the help of a registered dietician who has knowledge of the intuitive eating approach to recovery. This is the first step toward establishing a balanced relationship with food, as it helps you begin to reverse the eating-disorder process. For your safety, it is essential for you to work with both a physician and a registered dietitian with specialized training and experience in treating eating disorders. If you are not working with a physician and a dietitian already, start as soon as possible. Now you are mobilizing knowledgeable individuals, not your eating disorder, to help you with your nutrition.

Without regular nutrition, your body, thinking, emotional resilience, mood, judgment, energy, and motivation all become compromised. You may be unable to see it. I can see the effects of inadequate nutrition when a client regularly asks me to repeat the question I just asked, repeatedly forgets what we've discussed, or forgets what he or she has agreed to do. This usually disappears after nutrition is more stable and the brain is fed. Often my clients see the improvement in their thinking and agree (although not always in these words) that "malnutrition makes you stupid." This is one more reason why recovery, at this stage, needs to be about the food.

It is not unusual for clients to tell me that their bodies do not need regular nutrition because they have enough stored fat to keep them alive without eating anything at all for a year. You may notice a similar thought. You may also notice the urge to skip this section because you know as much about nutrition as any professional, and that structuring nutrition is important for others, but not for you. This is a common eating-disorder thought. I hear this from clients who are severely underweight, those who have been told by others that they are obese, and all weights in between. It is absolutely not true. *Always* be suspicious when your thoughts say that you are an exception to the rule, because such thoughts are serious eating-disorder tricks. It is a fact that malnutrition can occur at any weight. It is caused by deficits in micronutrients and hydration that cannot be diagnosed based on weight, size, the number of fat rolls you can pinch, or other criteria that you or your eating disorder come up with.

The first tier is the foundation upon which the other two tiers are built.

As part of our work to help you find a recovery strategy, we created, based on Robyn's work, our model for Nutritional Healing: A Three-Tier

Approach™. The first tier is the foundation upon which the other two tiers are built. This chapter teaches you about *Tier One: The Structured Approach*. For now, this is your most important tool as you build a foundation for your entire recovery. Start with the Structured Approach and stick with it until you can do it consistently despite your fear. Resist the urge (and your eating disorder's directive) to skip ahead to the next phase of eating because you "already know this stuff," or because you feel you should be further along, you're bored, you weigh enough anyway, or any other reason your eating disorder can create for doing so.

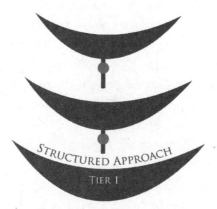

STRUCTURED APPROACH
TIER 1

NUTRITIONAL HEALING: A 3-TIER APPROACH™

Tier One: The Structured Approach

Eating Disorder: "You can't eat as much or as often as others." "You are small-boned and need less food than most people." Or "You are big-boned and can't eat as much food as most people because you will be fat." Or "You need to eat less often, not more regularly."

Truth: Notice how manipulative the eating disorder is? It actually uses opposing arguments to prove the same point, which is that you need to eat less than "normal." You would laugh at me if I tried that! Either way, you might be convinced that structured eating is wrong for you and will make you fat. It isn't true. One factor involved here is metabolism, which is one of our body's most brilliant survival mechanisms.

Perhaps you feel you are ready to eat "normally" and independently of your eating disorder's directives. Know that your eating disorder is desperate for you to experiment with eating "normally." Then it can convince you that you are eating adequately when you are following its mandates instead. To recover, you will need awareness, mental strength, and stamina in order to identify the eating disorder's voice. To build these, you need regular nutrition. You need to follow the structured plan and not a plan of your own (or your eating disorder's) design.

Structured eating is also important because your body and your mind may be unable to give you accurate signals about when to eat and what foods you need. Like Robyn, without structure, you enter the eating disorder's life-destroying cycle, and structure moves you away from that cycle. Restricting food makes you feel physically and psychologically deprived. Hunger and deprivation lead to bingeing. Bingeing leads to purging or increased efforts to restrict. The cycle is vicious, and it is a prescription for hopelessness.

Dietitians tend to recommend regular nutritional intake that includes at least three meals per day, as well as snacks, spaced fairly evenly throughout the day. Waiting more than three to four hours between meals or snacks can create fluctuations in the body's store of chemicals like serotonin, which gives us a sense of well-being, and blood sugar, which gives us energy. People often report things like "fuzzy" or "foggy" thinking, feeling grumpy, feeling tired, and other symptoms when their nutritional intake is inadequate or too infrequent.

Because eating disorders love to use eating between meals as an invitation to binge, let me clarify the purpose and the meaning of snacks. Snacks are small portions of food for the purpose of "topping off" your body's fuel tank to keep you functioning mentally, emotionally, and physically at your best. Sometimes you may feel hungry, sometimes you may feel full. If it isn't your body feeling uncomfortable with this, it will be your mind. That is just the way it is in early recovery. Be prepared to experience and endure these short-term symptoms to get through to the other side. Do not let your eating disorder distort my recommendation for topping off your tank by encouraging you to binge or omit eating. Typical snack ideas include jerky, granola, fruit, or an individual package of nuts.

At the beginning of Robyn's recovery she found it too overwhelming and difficult to snack, however over time she chose a "safe snack" by sticking to eating a piece of fruit at each allocated time. This snacking approach for Robyn kept her from feeling even more overwhelmed with eating. Robyn found that each time she kept her commitment to eat a regular snack she moved a little further from her eating disorder. Your dietitian can give you examples of snacks that might work best for you.

Throwing away ideas of "right" or "wrong," "good" or "bad," or "forbidden" foods is in the best interest of your recovery.

For some people it is helpful to begin by measuring food, particularly when guided by a dietitian. For others, the eating disorder uses measuring and counting to keep them fixated on food. We can tell you this: throwing away ideas of "right" or "wrong," "good" or "bad," or "forbidden" foods is in the best interest of your recovery.

We are giving you the formula Robyn ultimately used to structure her own nutrition for recovery. Robyn's plan worked best for her because it created a clear boundary for her eating disorder. And although it didn't tell her what she had to eat, it kept the eating disorder contained within its structure while it provided Robyn freedom to make choices of her own. Robyn says this safety net was her "structure for freedom."

Robyn used the Structured Approach to guide her food choices for a year, as she was afraid of making too many choices, and it helped to have the safety net. In addition, it was well beyond that year when she actually lost her fear of food. Robyn and I felt there needed to be some kind of tool to help relieve this added burden for those working on nutritional healing as part of their recovery. Let's face it, recovery is hard enough without adding the confusion of having no idea what foods to eat, how to distribute foods, or how to portion them. We consulted government sites and I talked with my dietitian colleagues, but we couldn't find a tool that we believe represents the range of nutritional choices and recommended portions without promoting anti-recovery concepts of "good" or "bad" foods. To visualize this is hard. That's why we developed our plate, Make Peace with Your Plate®, as a tool to help you use in our Structured Approach to eating. Take this tool to a registered dietitian who specializes in treating eating disorders. Ask your dietitian to consider your specific needs and help you customize a structured eating plan that works best for you.

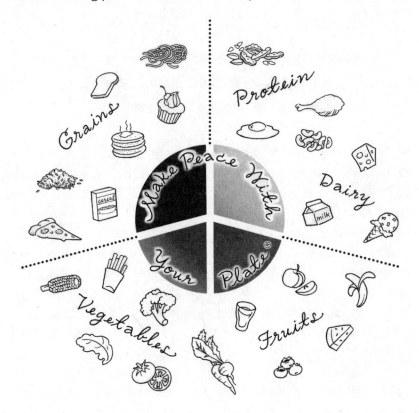

For additional help with using the Structured Approach to eating, some have used plates that we have imprinted with the above image. Those can be found on our website: www.robynandespra.com.

As we worked to create this guide for you, Robyn talked about the way she had to approach this tool in order for it to work in her own recovery. She recognized that her eating disorder was lurking close by, waiting to use this very tool to manipulate her thoughts and behaviors back toward her illness.

> "One of the things I needed to be conscious of was my willingness to play honestly come meal time. I needed to allow myself permission to eat what I felt like, filling the plate without judgment. I had to continually remind myself why I had the plate and not to abuse, manipulate, or make up a story of why I didn't have to stick to the structure. Piling food on the plate was as dishonest as not filling it."

 Use your own structured food plan that you and your dietitian create. Make a one-day sample schedule of how you might structure your own eating plan for recovery. (For example, don't plan breakfast at seven if you get up at ten.) Allow your times to vary if needed, but most importantly practice your structured food plan with realistic expectations of yourself, while also pushing enough so your eating disorder doesn't call the shots. This is about successful steps toward your recovery. When your eating disorder screams at you, locate your reasons to recover that you wrote down from Chapter One, and talk back.

Example:

Time	Helpful Hints
Breakfast 7:30 a.m.	Be flexible: If you wake up at 9:30 a.m., eat your breakfast then. Remember to eat three meals a day. Don't let your eating disorder trick you into starting with a snack, then only fitting in two meals.
Snack 10:00 a.m.	Set your snack time for a regular work or class break if you can. Otherwise, problem-solve how you can set aside a couple of minutes to eat or how to snack on-the-go.
Lunch 1:00 p.m.	Again, be flexible, and be sure to eat a meal, not a snack.

Time	Helpful Hints
Snack 3:30 p.m.	Again, you may need to problem-solve how to fit this in.
Dinner 7:00 p.m.	A high-risk time for bingeing or restricting! Freedom: You don't have to hide because of eating-disorder behavior anymore. Structure where and when you prepare food and eat if this is your high-risk time for bingeing or restricting. It is less likely that you will engage in these behaviors if you are not alone.
Snack 9:30 p.m.	Freedom: Most folks are hungry before bed. Having a snack now defies the eating-disorder rule that "you can't eat after a certain time of day because it will make you fat." Eat a snack anyway.

• •

To this day Robyn still returns to her structured eating foundation from time to time. Robyn maintains that her willingness to reset her nutrition to structured eating over and over again when she feels overwhelmed is a part of the key to her recovery.

Variety Is the Key

Eating Disorder: "Variety. That's a bunch of crap. The first bite of cheesecake you add to their *variety* plan will blow everything because you will lose control and never stop eating. The structure you really need is mine, not theirs."

Truth: Eating a variety of foods creates fuel that your body and brain need to maximize their capabilities.

Robyn included grains, fruits and vegetables, protein, and fats in every meal. This is necessary for healing, and it will automatically happen when you increase your range of foods. This also helps fuel your spirit, as each time you refuse to let the eating disorder decide what you will and won't eat, the less power it has over you.

It is important to create boundaries for your eating disorder in order to decrease its control over you. A vital function of working with a dietitian is to help you identify and normalize foods that trigger your eating-disorder behaviors, like those you fear and avoid as well as those you embrace and consume excessively or in an unbalanced way. Simultaneously, you must create freedom for yourself, so that neither you nor your eating disorder feels totally controlled or totally out of control. The force of will you expend trying to control your eating disorder through willpower alone is admirable, but burns a lot of mental and emotional energy, with limited and short-lived results. Save some energy for problem-solving and for keeping your behaviors on target.

Freedom exists within the boundaries. Begin fighting the disorder by using your ability to out-maneuver it, rather than using only willpower to control it. Control, when used by itself and without a clearly defined, objective plan, causes you to end up pushing against an eating disorder that is pushing back even harder. In the big picture, it gets you nowhere.

The freedom that you are seeking is the true power that is buried deep within you. Structured eating will help you begin to uncover that power as you define your own preferences rather than being controlled by those of the eating disorder. Whether you are rigid or experimental at certain times is your choice. And you win either way, because you either challenge an eating disorder food rule, or you challenge rigidity by making your own choice.

Inside of these boundaries, Robyn's freedom came through being able to make her own choices. Robyn allowed herself to sometimes choose the extremes because she knew either way she was still within the structure, but also challenged herself to choose from a middle path within the extremes—the places that she never usually visited within her illness. If she felt particularly frightened, instead of skipping the meal due to fear, she went with foods that felt safer (rice instead of a donut, for instance). When she felt more liberated or needed to challenge the eating disorder "rules," she went with food choices that felt more risky or rebellious (like fried chicken). It was her choice, and that was important to her, as it is to all of us. That is freedom. That is recovery.

What practical issues might get in the way of your structured food plan working? Make a list of these. Think of ways to solve the problems that might get in the way. Then write the solution you choose. Use it, and see if it works. If it works, good. If not, try another solution (and then another) until you find one that does work. Make a list of available foods to eat at those times. (Don't forget portable foods for when you are away from home.) Examples of issues that might need problem-solving include forgetting to eat or not having food with you when you need it.

There is freedom for creativity here, and I have seen amazingly creative solutions. For example, 1) Both Robyn and I have difficulty eating solid foods early in the morning. We both drink smoothies and shakes (not low-calorie or those designed for weight loss) that combine all food categories from the plate for breakfast (not *every* meal). 2) Sometimes activities get in the way of lunch. Honor your lifestyle. Set a lunchtime alarm on the phone; keep durable and portable foods in a bag, backpack, or your car so you can eat something no matter what.

Exercise

Eating Disorder: "Your body needs at least three hours of intense exercise a day or you'll be out of shape and flabby."

Truth: Exercise is to eating disorder recovery what fertilizer is to rose bushes. The right amount is helpful and too much is deadly. The right times and amounts of application are determined by specific criteria, not by how you feel (or instructions offered by an eating disorder).

> **It is important to talk with your physician and dietitian to determine how intensely and how long you should work out, as well as what types of exercise are safe for you. Ask your physician to tell you of any symptoms that might indicate you need to stop your exercise immediately. Follow your doctor's orders. Your eating disorder is not a doctor!**

Robyn limited herself to thirty to sixty minutes per day of exercise, as that approach worked well for her recovery. Absolutely refrain from any exercise that is driven by your eating disorder's need to burn calories, punish you, or control your activity in any other way.

Listen closely so you can catch your eating disorder's attempts to be in charge of this. If you find yourself arguing that there is a reason you should be doing more, know that this voice is most likely your eating disorder. Take a deep breath, clear your mind, and renegotiate your physician's and dietitian's guidelines with them as professionals, not with your eating disorder. For those who are inactive, it is important for you to safely add physical activity, as it decreases your vulnerability as well.

 Think of a physical goal that you want to work toward that is within the boundaries your healthcare providers have set for you. Then choose two physical activities that will help you work toward that goal. The best way to balance exercise for your recovery is to focus on "fun" activity goals.

Nutritional healing is the foundation upon which the rest of your recovery will be built. Do what you need to do, not because you are fearless, but because you refuse to let fear dictate your life.

> For life is good here where I stand.
> I am safe here where I stand.
> And there is no need for eating disorder,
> here where my feet meet the ground.

You have tried everything you can to control your eating disorder. It is safe for you to trust that you can and will have a better life without it. Today, put your trust in a new way of life where your body, mind, and soul are nurtured, where you look and feel your best—a magical place called recovery.

4.

Learning to Hit Curveballs

Eucalyptus Drops and the Bogeyman Within

By Robyn

One at a time, I took in the taste and texture of the eucalyptus drop, and each time my tongue rolled over the hardened lump, memories of childhood life oozed out, along with the sweetness of sugar and sharpness of eucalyptus. My brother Anton sent me a care package the other day filled with my favorite lollies. I felt like a little kid again. Yes, I still get giddy at the sight of my favorite candy. With the care package came a sense of opening up a treasure box of all the past events that made me who I am today. I find myself in curiosity now, instead of pain and regret, but still trying to connect the dots of my story, as if I may now be able to discover the reasons behind my circumstances.

Children are born with their own traits, mixed into their environment and later baked within their personalities throughout their lives. Each child takes away beliefs, skills, and ways of making sense of the world from his or her experiences. I am no exception. My mum's scent, the softness of her hands, the sound of her contagious giggle are forever imprinted in my heart like a butterfly's sense of direction—clear, without doubt, and with a true sense of knowing. For me, she was like deep breathing to anxiety, calming and medicinal. She was my soul supporter, encouraging my dreams and passions. She supported me, as me. I was her baby, even far into adulthood.

My dad, a good man, is a truck driver with a robust exterior and a beautiful heart that carries much heaviness and pain. Nearly seventy years old now, you can still find him on the highways between Sydney and Queensland, thinking and dreaming as he hums along in his semitrailer, trying to get to the next location as fast as possible. My dad's life meaning and purpose drove him to work tirelessly to provide for us when we were children. Like many men his worth as a father and as a man depended on this. He filled the provider role well for us. At the same time, it often had him absent during my youth, as he slept during the day and drove at night. I saw more of his uniform shirts on the folding basket awaiting ironing than I did him.

He was raised in a strict religious family, to believe in and to fear the judgment of a condemning and punitive god. Wanting to protect us from emotional burdens such as guilt that he had experienced in his youth, he discarded the harsh and fearful boundaries imposed upon him in his childhood home and imposed few in ours. He profoundly loved us, and we him. As is so often the case in parenting, he could not know what he had not learned. He endeavored to create for us the opposite of his environment, but having no boundaries accidently caused its own version of pain for me, like the sense that I was responsible for things well beyond my capacity to control.

When Mum became ill with lupus, life stopped. My young brain searched for answers as my ever-present and loving mum was now behind closed doors, bedridden and fighting to stay alive. There was very little privacy in our home. I could often be found sitting on the toilet talking to my mum as she showered. So when her bedroom door closed, we understood it was a place we could not go. I wanted to. But I knew she was busy willing her body to live. Now the pain inside me, the pain that I always took to my mother, I was left with. Not knowing how to soothe myself, my mind was stuck, all alone.

I was never physically alone, but I felt the emotional isolation. All of us in the family dealt with this life change so very differently. My sister, Betty, left home before Mum became ill. She left at sixteen, was married by eighteen, and gave birth to her first child three months before her nineteenth birthday. My mum was a twenty-one-year-old single parent working in a pub in Liverpool when she met my dad. Dad immediately took to Betty like any father would his first-born; but later when a child of his own blood was born, Betty was unintentionally left in the background. She sought to soothe her resulting confusion and emotional pain with eating for hunger and for emotional comfort. To this day, some of our family's story is that her weight gain was caused by appendix surgery. Although I didn't see my sister much, it appeared that out of all of our family members my sister and I used similar coping patterns, one of those being the use of food.

The emotional dynamic of resentment and fear set the stage for conflict and chaos in our home. If it wasn't Betty and Dad screaming at each other, it was Mum and Dad. My brother Anton and I were bystanders. It was my relationship with Anton that helped me cope with the emotional upheavals. I experienced glimpses of feeling valued and worthwhile as I aided in the concoction of mindless boy games. I loved to hang out with my brother and his friends. Anton is twenty months older than me. I was grateful to be Anton's trustworthy assistant among his popular friends because I was unpopular, teased, and called "chubby" by my peers. I forgot all about that when I joined in on his riff-raff.

As I dealt with the anxiety within, Anton dealt with it by not dealing with it. One night as we lay in our beds in the darkness, I said to my brother, "Okay, if Mum and Dad separate, you go with Dad and look after him, and I'll go with Mum and look after her. Promise?"

"Shut up, Rob," he said. But he heard me. My brother always heard me.

There came a time where even with the eating disorder there was very little escape from my feelings. My emotions would blindside me like an avalanche. Without my even being aware, my thoughts would gain momentum, and my body would be caught in a whirlwind of sheer panic, sobs of desperation, and the sensation that I was the thing that was so very wrong. Not able to cope with the emotions rapidly taking over, I spun out of control. I would try to get up and fight, but as with any avalanche, fighting was useless. My emotions had already buried me.

It's taken many years to learn how to stop being blindsided emotionally. I still succumb to it on occasion. I just have more awareness now of the choices I have in participating. Most of the time, I get to choose what to do with my emotions and my recovery. Oh, I still get challenged by them. Believe me! I am human, fallible and breathing. I still feel very deeply, and sometimes that feels wonderful; but when it doesn't, and I don't want to be a part of it, I decide when and how I want to "press pause." I have come to believe that it is in our pauses that we get the opportunity to rewrite our story.

I met my husband, Tim, outside a twelve-step meeting. I had determined that quitting alcohol *first* was what I needed in order to find long-term recovery from my eating disorder, because the "fuck it" button that I pressed whenever I drank alcohol prevented me from being conscious of who I really wanted to be. The bottom line: When I drank, I would either go home with a man or a bag of food. In either case, the "mornings after" were rarely pretty for me. I have heard many stories of others with eating disorders who did not have to stop drinking alcohol, and their recovery is full. But my "switching the witch for the bitch" is a constant.

I spotted Tim from across the room. I always knew that I was waiting for someone, but never knew what that someone would be like. When I spotted Tim, I knew he was the one I was waiting for. Sounds corny, I know. Nine years my senior with wit, humor, charisma, and looks that made me drool, he was trouble. And I loved it.

Tim and I are two very passionate people. I love him to bits, madly, deeply. When we argue I can still manage to become as confused as that little girl struggling to understand her emotions as I faced my mother's closed bedroom door. The need to fix the problem so I could get out of the discomfort has led me to further avalanches I might have bypassed had I paused, taken a breath, and really grasped what was going on.

Tim often travels out of state for work. He is a recovery support specialist who intervenes with addicts and later reintegrates them into their home life after treatment. With our girls getting older—Chloe is five and a half and Lilly is seven—they recognize their dad's absence, and he, theirs, so we Skype nightly when he is away. One particular night, just before I called the girls over to talk to Tim at the computer, I told him about my day. I was excited, ignoring his low and drained energy, as I told him about the white trestle I had purchased online. I planned to put an old door that I had refurbished and glass panel on top of it to form a desk. I thought I only needed one trestle to go under the middle of the door, so when Tim asked me if I had purchased an additional trestle to go on the other end of it, I said no. He lashed out: "What do you mean? Didn't you buy another one?" I felt stupid. I was baffled by his reaction and also by the new awareness that I would, in fact, require *two* trestles, and the interaction quickly became uncomfortable. I asked Tim to stop speaking to me as he was, and he told me I was being defensive. I recognized in that moment that it was his emotions that were stronger than the situation warranted. With this clarity, I was able to react with a calm voice, without escalating the situation. The fact was, he was lonely (missing his girls painfully) and tired, which appeared to influence his interaction with me, and I recognized this. My choices were to engage anyway or step back for a while. *That time* I chose to step back.

For the record, I usually, most of the time even, yell back at Tim, defending myself with a vengeance. I feel challenged and reactive. But on that day, I simply got off the computer without cursing and sat with my girls on the sofa as they watched TV. I sorted through all my emotions until I reached my truth, wading through the usual feeling of worthlessness and the thoughts that came with it: *You're a bad person. It's all your fault. He's tired for goodness sake.* I didn't allow myself to be swept up in all that, however. I've learned to recognize when I have spoken or acted in a way that I am not okay with; I get a sense in my gut that tells me so. I didn't get that feeling on that night. In my stillness, I got a sense that Tim already had hard feelings hitting him that were separate from me. Although his words were directed at me, I was clear it was not all about me, and the damn trestle!

The truth is we are all human; I forget this sometimes, especially when my emotions are high. Still, it can be uncomfortable for me to sit with myself or not move into self-doubt when there is nothing to be immediately fixed. *I'm being too harsh; maybe I should just ask him what's really going on. No*, I told myself. *Allow it to just be, and do not put any more energy into it tonight.* So I did not allow myself to obsess about it for the rest of the night, but simply breathed instead as I cuddled up with my daughters.

It turns out my feelings won't kill me. If I sit with my intense emotions, they will not swallow me up, make me go crazy, or cause something catastrophic to happen to me. It turns out that my reactions are the bogeyman in life, not that I have a broken mind. You see, just as my mum got to choose a different lifestyle to place her lupus into remission, I now have the choice to change my lifestyle by facing all the pain that I have based many of my decisions, behaviors, and reactions upon, and find another way that betters my life and the lives of all those around me. My mum, too, taught me this from behind closed doors.

What to Do When the Bogeyman Jumps Out

By Espra

Eating Disorders Love Curveballs

Eating Disorder: "You blew that one. You really can't handle anything, can you? You're lucky I'm here. At least there's hope for you to be competent at something."

Truth: The anesthetic benefits of addictive behaviors wear off quickly and your emotions flood back with a renewed vengeance. Nothing about this devastating pattern helps you learn to cope better. It only makes you better at using eating-disorder behaviors.

You probably already feel vulnerable, maybe even fragile and out of control, due to the river of emotions that floods through you. Then life throws you a surprise, good or bad, that you didn't see coming and the eating disorder tells you that you are defective because you handled it "wrong." You are convinced that everyone else handles things right and that something is wrong with you if you strike out. Do you see the lie? No matter how you handle life's curveballs, you risk becoming racked with even more guilt, shame, and fear than before.

How do you cope with emotions that are so intensely painful that it seems they will consume you? The eating disorder readily hands you a solution. The distractions brought by eating-disorder thinking or the comfort delivered through eating-disorder behaviors might seem like the perfect solutions for coping with pain. But they will only leave you at the mercy of the same destructive illness that is threatening your long-term peace and happiness.

The key to increasing your ability to cope with life's curveballs is—just as Robyn did in her interaction with Tim—to notice what is happening, find a pause button, and push it. Pausing and shutting down are two different things. Robyn recognized that, more than Tim's mind, his emotions were driving his speech. She also recognized feeling blindsided by her own emotions. Robyn's automatic thoughts and physical sensations warned her that her all-too-familiar avalanche of shame, fear, and anger was coming toward her with dizzying speed and force. Of course it mattered that Robyn felt and honored the sting of the pain she felt from Tim's words. And it mattered that Robyn quickly pushed a pause button before her emotions took over and yelled back at Tim "with a vengeance." That's what emotions do when they run unchecked. Robyn exited the conversation (she insists that she didn't even use the "f" word) to allow her intense emotions, physical sensations, and thoughts to settle. It was only after her pause that Robyn could see her "I deserved that" thoughts as more of a byproduct of her shame than a fact.

Robyn knew it was important to pause, both physically and mentally, putting her focus elsewhere and simply breathing for the night. If Robyn had mentally continued the conversation with Tim during her "pause," her emotions would have grown stronger. Instead of helping, the pause would have merely delayed her giving Tim an earful. Always remember, the heart of pausing is to get your attention *away* from obsessing and ruminating about the situation by placing your full attention on what you are doing in the moment. The purpose for pausing is not to ignore or dishonor your feelings. That is dangerous. Pausing is about creating enough space from the situation to keep your emotions from making the decisions about how you act, robbing you of your own choices and authentic control.

Only through years of working to build her ability to pause has Robyn come to learn that feelings won't kill her, and, although sometimes painful, they are not bad in and of themselves. Only after settling her shame and fear could Robyn use her awareness to respect her emotions about the situation at hand. Then, armed with her authentic power, Robyn could decide how to deal with the situation in a way that maintained her self-respect by honoring her feelings as well as her needs.

It is when emotions dictate your thoughts and behaviors that you can quickly strike out; foul things up; and get thrown out of places, situations, and relationships altogether. It is this even darker place that feels like death to many.

The risk with eating disorders and addictive behaviors in general is that obsessing about and acting on eating-disorder thoughts and urges can be your way of "pushing pause." This is not pausing. It is unplugging and shutting down. Shutting down electronic devices usually restores them to default settings. When you have an eating disorder, your default settings are obsessing about your body, food, eating, not eating, exercise, purging, counting calories, and (fill in the blank). Obsessing left alone leads to acting. For example, many of my clients find themselves standing in front of a mirror, staring and poking at their bodies with disgust, more frequently and for longer periods of time when they are already upset. These are the times when you might find yourself not caring about recovery at all, much less your reasons for pursuing recovery. This is why an intentional and more skillful, non-eating-disordered pause is needed. This chapter is devoted to teaching you how to pause.

Curveballs Catch Us All Off Guard

Eating Disorder: "Of course Robyn couldn't cope. She was young, and she had *real* problems. You, on the other hand, have no reason to have trouble coping with your life."
Truth: Being human comes with problems; and problems, big or small, can be painful. Do you turn to eating-disorder thoughts or behaviors as your coping strategy in difficult times? If so, does it appear to be a truly effective coping strategy in the long run? Think about this some more. It is probably more of a numbing strategy, which is not at all helpful in the long-term.

I don't know much about baseball. I do know that sometimes it seems like everything in our lives is a curveball—elusive, confusing, and just beyond our reach. We think we've got it figured out, then it changes its course right before our eyes, without warning. My clients frequently ask why this happens to them. Wise people over the ages have responded to this universal question in many philosophical ways. My response is, "I don't know. I just know that's the way it is." Suffering is a human condition, not—as the eating disorder would have you believe—an affliction reserved for "unworthy, undisciplined, fat people who are disgusting and need to be punished" (these are eating disorder words, not mine). Sometimes we can see curveballs coming, but most of the time we cannot. We often end up wishing we had managed things differently.

Somehow, you have to figure out how to survive curveballs without running to an eating disorder or other addictive behaviors. You also have to refrain from living in fear that everything coming your way is a curveball. Overestimating the probability of a catastrophic outcome may seem like a way to protect yourself, but it's actually a formula for increasing anxiety, misery, and suffering. You need protective measures that will not take you out of the batter's box or remove you from the game altogether. When you feel like dealing with life and recovery is just not your game, take a time out; then return to the game and do your best to muddle through, even if you are sure you've already lost. That's the way we all have to do it. That's a big part of recovery.

Overestimating the probability of a catastrophic outcome may seem like a way to protect yourself, but it's actually a formula for increasing anxiety, misery, and suffering.

For many people, Robyn included, early learning environments and relationships are affected by illness, other traumas, or merely the inability of caregivers to use or teach coping skills. Keep in mind that individuals with eating disorders are biologically predisposed to high levels of emotional sensitivity, thus more intense emotion. This is where the combination of genetics and learning environment come together to get in the way of acquiring coping skills earlier in life. Needing to learn so many of these concrete skills later in life and in a more condensed time frame can make putting them into action feel slow, tedious, and overwhelming. The good news is that with learning, time, and practice, it is possible.

Keep Your Eye on the Ball

Eating Disorder: "Exactly. If you keep your focus on me there's no way you can go wrong."

Truth: When you keep your eye on eating-disorder thoughts and behaviors, you can't miss what they drive you to see. But you will miss many other important things around you.

I hope you made a list in Chapter One of your reasons to recover and the harm of embracing your eating disorder, even at difficult times. (Sorry. Recovery won't happen if you bargain that taking the eating disorder out of the closet to get you through hard times and tucking it neatly away when things are smooth is good enough.) Commit to reading your list when things get hard and *before* you act. Reading your list will help you take a step back. If it stops the behaviors, that is progress. If it doesn't, you will need to keep using additional skills that are presented in this chapter.

Respect What Is

In order to face extremely difficult emotions without running for the distraction or illusion of control found in obsessive thoughts and addictive behaviors, you must first acknowledge that something has happened and that you are suffering terribly because of it. You might want it to be different, but you must respect that in that moment it is not the way you want it to be. I am not pushing you to like what is happening, be happy about it, think happy thoughts, say things are okay, or stop hoping or working for change. Genuine acceptance is the first step in seeing and responding to a situation as it actually is. Otherwise you might gather a hose to fight a fire when it is a flood that is threatening your house.

It helps to come up with a meaningful statement that helps get your mind focused on first accepting that a difficult situation has shown up. I teach my clients a three-sentence approach to help with this:

I want _____. I wish I had _____.

But I don't. For example: *I want that one true person in my life who loves me. I wish I had that one true person in my life who loves me. But right now, I don't.*

One of my clients told me this set of statements, "Drops me right into validating my wants, my wishes, and respecting and accepting that what I've got in this moment is something different. Bam, it drops me right into looking at what I need to do with what is actually happening in my world right now. It's like then I can do something useful." Another acceptance statement I often hear people use is, "It is what it is." The words you choose are not as important as finding some way to pull your mind away from how things "should" be, or who caused them, and toward respecting what is actually happening. Only then can you decide how to effectively approach it.

 What statement can you create that is meaningful to you, and that will help you respect what has shown up for you? Will you work with one of those above or find another one that resonates for you? Write it down. Commit it to memory.

After you drop yourself into the reality of what is going on, there are a few things you can do to carry that acceptance forward. Warning: Reading this information and saying your statement one time does not glue you to your acceptance decision. You will need the additional bonding power of a strong adhesive. The way to strengthen the bonding power is through repetition. Over and over, you will need to affirm your statement, take a deep breath, let it out, relax your body, uncross your arms, relax your hands, and turn your palms up in a gesture of allowing in information beyond what is rocking around in your mind and body. As you open your body, remind yourself of your decision to respect and work effectively with what this moment has brought to you.

Your alternative is to cross your arms, furrow your brow, clench your fists, stomp your feet, and say the eating disorder's favorite words: "I won't (or I can't)." We tend to do this when things are not going our way. Refusing to tolerate pain when things are not going our way is much easier than working to respect and accept the reality; however, it gets in the way of getting through the difficulty with a sense of dignity and self-respect. It gets in the way of recovery.

Be prepared to use your statement as your path to return your mind again and again to your decision to accept instead of push away what is presenting itself to you in the moment. Then gather information so you can decide the most helpful next step. Practice, repeat, and don't expect to perfect this process. It is in the mere practice of reminding ourselves of our ultimate choice, our intention, to accept one difficult moment at a time and repeatedly reopening our body and mind to the intention of that misery. Over time, it can become a little less miserable.

Body Mechanics

Once you've decided to tolerate hard emotions long enough to keep yourself from doing the things that will make matters worse in the long run, you can begin using other skills to help you ride out emotional and behavioral urges instead of acting on them. Although it might feel that without an outlet, the urges will continue to build forever—believe it or not, these emotions and urges eventually decrease if you don't act on them. It will be difficult for you to believe that right now, so please trust me. The only way to build faith in this is to give it a good, honest, lengthy try for yourself and see what you notice.

Because turning to behaviors that quickly numb emotion brings significant relief immediately, it sets up a powerful reinforcement cycle that is difficult to break. The package is wrapped so attractively that it is tough to resist. Please work hard to resist it anyway.

Tolerating pain by using skills, on the other hand, takes more time and effort but helps you forego the behaviors that make matters worse. However, you may not feel better or relieved. Learning to tolerate the pain helps decrease your chances of running to eating-disorder behaviors in a panic. In the long run, you will see the benefits of using coping skills over numbing your mind. My clients appreciate the sense of pride, authentic power, and self-respect that emerge from those deeper places within as they practice over time. Stick with it.

This is a dangerous time to let your emotions have a mind of their own. Take some time for the dust to settle. Give yourself time to look at the situation you are in with eyes and a mind that are open and able to take in new information. This sort of mindful, aware, and awake state is often compared to turning on the lights in a dark room.

Pay attention to the sensations in your body. This is not to be confused with paying attention to what you think about your body or what you see when you look at your body. If you notice your intense emotions include rapid heart rate, shortness of breath, dizziness, rapid thoughts, tension, or other physical signals, this means that your body has invoked its powerful fight or flight response. Your sympathetic nervous system has primed your body for action and it is time to change your body mechanics. In order to cope with intense emotion, assuming you do not need to fight or flee for your life, it is helpful to intentionally activate your parasympathetic system, which is responsible for how your body functions when it is not in danger or is at rest. Just like rebooting a computer, there are ways to reboot your body. Slowing down your body clears the way for your brain to get unlocked from the intense emotion (what is going on inside of you) and focus on what is going on around you. Getting information about what is going on around us as well as inside of us positions us to develop a course of action, or at least our next helpful step.

The next few skills can be used to physically reset your body by activating your parasympathetic nervous system, at those times when your sympathetic nervous system has unnecessarily taken over. These skills, along with many other skills in this chapter, are described in more detail in the Resources section at the back of this book, where you will also find recommendations on how to find additional information and help.

Breathing Techniques

It is hard to breathe when our emotions are high. Many of my clients report an increase in their anxiety when they feel intense emotion that makes it hard to breathe and someone says, "Take a deep breath." They are trying to breathe but can only gasp for air and get in small amounts, which makes them hyperventilate and become more anxious. (Hyperventilation and anxiety have many symptoms in common.) If this happens to you, use the *How to Take a Deep Breath* technique explained in the Resources section.

As soon as you can get air in, focus on making your breaths slower, deeper, and more even, with a slightly longer exhale than inhale. You will need to practice this until you can do it automatically. You are overriding your body's basic survival instinct by breathing deeply and evenly when you are angry, afraid, or sad, and that does not happen easily.

Making your breathing deeper, slower, and more regular is one of the most effective strategies for reducing emotional arousal and distress fast.

I teach two specific styles of breathing, *deep breathing* and *paced breathing,* because they have been shown to be the most effective at quickly lowering intense emotion. Paced breathing shows promising results with rapidly decreasing anxiety and takes only about one minute to complete. Deep breathing can take two to five minutes to reboot your body and can be more difficult to use in times of distress, but some people prefer it. Instructions to help you learn both styles of breathing can be found in the Resources section, and I encourage you to experiment with each style to learn what is helpful to you.

Also, a daily twenty-minute deep breathing practice is beneficial in decreasing high emotion into the next day and will have a cumulative effect of decreased anxiety over time. Simply by taking regular, deep, full breaths throughout the day, you can improve your emotional, mental, and physical well-being and resilience.

 Experiment with breathing styles. Choose a way to try each of them long enough to become familiar with it. Play with each one until you find a length of time (in seconds) that is comfortable for you to breathe in, pause, and breathe out for a bit longer. What numbers work best for you for paced breathing and what numbers work best for you for deep breathing? You will begin to get a sense that you prefer one over the other to help you settle your body. Choose which one you would like to use as your emergency skill, write it down, and continue to practice it regularly.

When your body and emotions wind up, you can sit down right there, right then, regulate your breathing, and decrease the intensity of your emotions. You can take these breathing techniques anywhere you go! How cool is that? Now we're talking real control.

Progressive Muscle Relaxation

Progressive muscle relaxation (PMR) was developed in the 1920s by a physician named Edmund Jacobson. Jacobson hypothesized that anxiety and stress lead to muscle tension, which, in turn, increases painful emotions. When the body is in a relaxed state, there is little muscle tension, leading to decreased intensity in feelings of stress, fear, anxiety, and anger. Your breathing and heart rate slow down and your blood pressure decreases. Is this sounding familiar? He concluded that by learning how to relax muscle tension, a person can decrease the intensity of their emotions.

PMR is done by tensing and relaxing muscle groups, in a sequence, throughout the body. Each muscle group is purposefully tensed and then released for a few seconds before continuing on to the next muscle group. Instructions to help you learn progressive muscle relaxation can also be found in the section on Resources.

It helps to use a numerical scale of one to ten or one to one hundred (subjective units of distress scale or SUDS) to measure how big the emotion is before and after using each skill. This will help you get an idea of what is happening in between "I can't stand this" and "feeling all better," because either extreme is rare. Several skills are often needed, back to back, to get the emotion to a manageable level. It also helps you learn which skills are more and less helpful in reducing your difficult emotions.

With practice, you can learn how to effectively lower the intensity of your emotions. Many of my clients also use a combination of breathing and relaxation techniques to help them fall asleep at night or when they wake up and cannot get back to sleep.

Being On Guard versus Being in Control

Eating Disorder: "Since you can't handle hard things, always be on the lookout. Never let your guard down and cut pain off at the pass. That's how to stay in control."

Truth: If you don't swing, you may be less likely to strike out. You also will never get a base hit, much less a home run. The eating disorder says that intentionally "failing" will allow you to maintain some control. Actually, failing on your own terms gives you absolutely no control—and takes away your chances of having anything more. (I know, I know . . . at least you don't have far to fall when a risk doesn't work out.) Think about that. Exactly what is it that you have control over when you intentionally fail? The question is do you want to spend the rest of your life sitting in a grave to assure that you never fall into a hole and hurt yourself?

The eating disorder wants you to believe that it helps you avoid fear, embarrassment, and pain. If you don't swing at curveballs and instead throw down the bat and walk away, it might seem like you can hold on to more dignity than if you swing and miss, strike out, and suffer the embarrassment of failure in front of everyone. Eating-disorder thinking can lead you to believe that taking risks will result in a bigger fall than you can tolerate.

Are you willing to consider a change from avoiding curveballs to learning how to identify them sooner and face them? Would you consider trying to muster some skills to help you stay in the game? It's difficult. If you practice and use the skills in this chapter over and over, you'll have your armor ready and your tools cared for and polished—and you will be more likely to take them up and use them when necessary. If you stay with this strategy, bits of hope, confidence, and trust in yourself will begin to, almost imperceptibly, show up. You can't change the fact that a curveball has been thrown your way, but you can learn to see it for what it is and do something that will help address the problem instead of making matters worse.

So, okay. The curveball is in front of you. You have decided to respect that it is, indeed, a curveball—you hate it, you are shaking in your cleats, and you don't want any part of it. Ultimately you want this to go differently, because the way you've always done it hasn't worked out so well. You use breathing to relax your body and willingly open your hands so you can decide what to do and what will be effective. You remind yourself that what you've got in the moment is what you've got for the moment. You use one or two of the previously listed skills, which bring the intensity of the emotion down some. You know your thoughts are good at tumbling around in your mind and bringing in more distress. Your job here is to add additional skills and continue to use them until your emotions seem to stabilize enough for you to think a little more clearly. What now?

Pause
Eating Disorder: "There is no better way to get off of a spinning merry-go-round than to hang out with me."
Truth: It is true that getting lost in eating-disorder thoughts and/or behaviors makes the chaos of things whirling around you disappear. The problem is that the merry-go-round hasn't actually stopped. You just closed your eyes.

I often teach my clients to use the word "pause" to help them remember to
1. push pause,
2. step away, until the dust settles,
3. see the big picture, and
4. engage in life.

Grounding Skills
These skills can help you pause and turn your attention elsewhere while you let things cool off a bit. They involve both the body and the mind. Identify the skills that might be useful to you based on what seems to fit or intrigue you. Stay away from comparing or thinking about what is "normal," "weird," or what you think you "should" or "should not" do. Individualize these skills, experiment with them, and make them your own so they can help you. When you need them, stick with them, doing

one after another, until you can think well enough to make real choices instead of doing the same old emotionally driven behaviors that bring you the same old results.

Do Something

Watch videos; do puzzles; go to a movie; knit; clean the house; go for a drive; play an instrument; play with a dog; call or visit a friend (talk about something other than the problem); play games; practice a random act of kindness; make something for someone; send cards, jokes, inspirational texts, or messages; babysit to give a parent a break; visit, entertain, or read to residents in a nursing home; visit someone who is lonely; run errands for someone in need. Engage your mind with word, math, or logic puzzles; count backward from 100 by seven; play alphabet games; remember the birthdates of people in your life; count tiles on the floor; or count circles or squares in the room. Try something that is mindless for you but that holds your attention like a magazine or book. Encourage yourself like you would cheerlead a friend by saying, "I can do this. I can do it differently this time. I'll do it one step at a time." Many people think that if they are worthy and loved enough, there will be others around to encourage them. That is not necessarily the case. What's that saying? "If you want something done right, you've got to do it yourself." Encouragement is one of those things. Anything you get from others is a bonus and a gift to appreciate.

Jiggle the emotion loose with activities that bring up a different feeling like inspiring or funny videos or movies; upbeat, empowering, or calming music; funny, peaceful, or inspirational photos; or reading jokes or inspirational quotes. Burp (yes, I'm serious) or do something playful. Experiment with using various activities to learn what provokes different emotions for you.

Spiritual practices like talking to a higher power or deity, reading or reciting scripted poems or prayers such as the Serenity Prayer or the Rosary, chanting, meditation, metta phrases, and many others can help decrease painful emotions.

Warning: Don't fall for the eating disorder's suggestions of going for a run or getting ice cream. Find activities that work for you, but are not destructive, addictive, risky, or give eating-disorder thoughts or behaviors any room to show up. Throw yourself completely into them. Your imagination is your only limitation. There is no need to box yourself in. Just make sure you don't use behaviors that suck you into checking out or shutting down to the degree that you avoid versus re-enter your life. Remember, the way to use skills to improve your ability to cope with curveballs in the long run is to pause, not shut down. That said, if you can find something to hold your attention, that is legal, that is not harmful to others or yourself, go for it.

Wait, Wait, Wait . . .

At the amusement park near where I grew up, they wanted us to stay seated on rides until they stopped completely. The attendants would say, "Wait . . . wait . . . hold on . . . hold it . . . hold it . . . now get out!" It was their way of making sure everyone waited until it was safe to exit. To do otherwise presented unnecessary danger. So it is with emotions. As you are learning, in crisis times it takes a lot of holding on and a lot of "wait, wait, waits" to keep from prematurely unbuckling your seatbelt and jumping into trouble.

Use Your Senses

Robyn's mom soothed her when Robyn was sad or scared until, way too soon, her mom couldn't and Robyn was sometimes left trying to soothe her pain by herself. Restricting nutrition, obsessing about calories, bingeing and purging, etc. all can provide the temporary function of soothing.

One of the most helpful ways to soothe yourself without causing additional harm is to immerse yourself in the present moment, using your senses instead of thoughts about what has or what will occur. You can look at photos of loved ones (not someone you have lost) and beautiful places; notice what you see on a walk; look at your pet, a loved one, a child, or flowers and let what you see sink into your heart. Listen to music, relaxation CDs, and nature or other sounds that actually soothe you (more than those you think *should* soothe you). Touch a pet, a baby's hair, your own hair, or a favorite blanket; run your hand through a bowl of uncooked rice; use a heating pad; take a warm bath, using bubbles if you like the way they feel. Smell lotions, candles, coffee, hay, oils, and perfumes, but only those you really like. The sense of taste can be helpful for soothing, but due to the thoughts and emotions that can get wrapped up around food when an eating disorder is present, it's best just to leave your taste buds out of your toolkit for calming emotions.

Some people fall into soothing themselves more than they address difficulties in their lives and it causes bigger problems later on. Many people think they don't deserve to be soothed, or that others should soothe them. It is ultimately your job to soothe yourself when you need it, and help from others is a gift to be appreciated. What will work for you? Pay attention. Your body will tell you what it finds soothing.

 Look at the skills for tolerating intense and painful emotions in this chapter. Let them guide you in identifying four skills that might be helpful as a starting place. Use my examples or create your own. Experiment with them. Play around with them. See which ones hold your attention. As you try one skill at a time, use the zero-to-one-hundred scale to rate the intensity of your emotion before and after. (Even if you are not in crisis, you will still probably notice some decrease in negative mood and/or an increase in positive mood.)

Pausing gives you options to look beyond eating-disorder or other addictive behaviors to cope with crises. We all know that coping with intense emotions and difficult circumstances is probably part of an eating disorder's function in your life. So give yourself some choices. If you try a skill for a while and your difficult mood either doesn't decrease or, worse yet, it increases, chances are your mind is on the crisis and not on what you are doing in that moment. You might need to change to a different skill that occupies your mind. As you begin to endure emotional onslaughts in a more effective way, over time you will begin to see, like Robyn, that huge emotions do not swallow you up forever when you face them. Hang on tight and weather the storm. Although it can feel like you are drowning in emotion, the storm eventually passes and the flood recedes.

You may find yourself going back to eating-disorder behaviors to help you tolerate distress. Remember, recovery is turning your mind back to doing things differently and learning what you can about what went wrong before. It is like kicking dirt into the hole you keep falling into. With time, the hole will be less deep, causing less harm when you fall in, and allowing you to get out sooner. As you practice pressing pause, preventing harmful reactions, and then responding to difficult situations, you build and start to trust the very emotional strength and know-how that are needed to climb out of the trenches.

I am me,
with all my emotions, flaws, beauty, and life lessons.
None of them define me.
Yet all of them make me.

Today, I will honor all that I am in its full integrity.

5.
Catch the Liar Red-Handed

Chinese Food and the Hot Malibu Sun

By Robyn

It felt more like flying the coop than leaving home had. It was more painful than breaking up with a lover. It was like a war inside myself, and I was getting ready to go in and reclaim the territory that my illness had occupied for most of my life.

While I was ready to pull out the big guns and infiltrate the enemy, I was still plagued with fear coupled with a sense of sadness that I believed others couldn't understand unless they had been through it. It was like the pain you feel after losing a parent. Others can console and sympathize, but if they have never lost a parent, they just don't get it. This sadness had started to steep in me, and it was anything but a cup of tea. What was it? Was I sad because I was fighting the part of me that I had depended on to save me? Was it that the illness was also my companion? Was it that I wanted to be well, but feel beautiful to the world also, and didn't know if that was possible? Was I scared? Was it that by questioning my eating disorder, I was questioning the life I had wasted, and that I had to concede my own responsibility in that? It was all of that.

I was so attached to the lies. It was, after all, going against the grain to question my illness, which had become a part of my identity. There was no longer a line that set me apart from my illness. I was enmeshed, and it was I who had to start detangling myself from "it." I had noticed the lies of the illness. I saw them from the corner of my eye, and I chose to ignore them. I also understood that if I allowed myself to pause within these questioning moments, I would have to confront the lies. It was like going to get your purse and seeing someone you love with his hand in it. You know there is something amiss. I had to start confronting my illness by looking it in the metaphorical eyes and saying: "You have your hand in my purse. Is there a reason you have your hand on my property?" And when it provided its excuse (there is always an excuse), I had to state firmly: "There is no excuse for this behavior." Because there is never any excuse to steal, and my illness had stolen my life. Now I needed to step in and take back what was mine.

I found it most difficult to believe that others didn't judge me by my size. After all, I judged people by their size. I compared myself to others all the time, and found strength in being thinner and shame in being larger. I starved at people and ate at myself, a brutal punishment either way. My worth was invested in the way I looked, so why would people not judge me because of it? Just because I wanted to end the eating disorder didn't mean that I wanted to feel big and unattractive. I had and still have a desire to feel my best, to feel beautiful. I just had to accept that the way to get there was not the way I was going. My body was dying. My mind was closed to the world. I had to have faith that there was more to me, and indeed to my life, than my body. I knew that if I wanted to be rid of the eating disorder I had to be willing to reevaluate my need to control the world through my body.

At nineteen I had my first relationship with Dylan. Dylan hit me within a week of our first meeting after I had straddled him teasingly. There was no doubt that I was playing, and he shamed me with what I realize now was a vicious way to create an understanding of who was in control. Instead of leaving Dylan immediately, I rode my bicycle in the dark to buy Chinese food for him. I apologized for his behavior, just as I had apologized for so many wasted years for my illness's behavior. I protected his behavior and justified it by believing my own lack of worth.

I remember sitting on the steps at a movie theatre and Dylan telling me how fat I was. We had just had an argument, and he would not allow me to have what he considered the last word. He spat out at me, telling how his last girlfriend was a personal trainer and so much better looking than me. And right there I saw what I perceived as the true value of starving. It would be the weapon I would use to gain control. I became his accessory and dependent. While at times he begged me to eat, I believed he loved me more because I'd become a petite shell of a woman whom he now needed to look after. I played small so he could feel big, just like I did with my illness. The truth was I found love in playing small. To question that would have been to question my part in it and my fear that I was too much for others to handle. It would have demanded that I face who I really was and own it. Be it. Honor it. Only by doing that would I teach people how to treat me.

◆ ◆ ◆

One Sunday evening when I was sixteen, I opened the garage door and walked into the smoky, dark, rectangular room designed as a "man cave" for my father, a place he practically lived in. It was quiet with a sense of hopelessness. I was wearing my mother's pink satin pajamas. They made me feel comforted and slimmer, as they draped baggily on my frame.

My dad was sitting, staring at the wall as he always did, smoking as he always did. He was lost in a world of complete fantasy, so as to forget the dead marriage in which he lived. He glanced at the one thing he gave himself, a six-by-six-inch TV that was bolted to the same brick wall he stared at. He was bare-chested, his stomach rolling over his blue shorts that rode up to gather at the top of his thighs. He had not cared for himself or his appearance for quite some time.

He loved to hear me read my poetry, and I loved feeling pride when I heard his response to it. As I stood beside him, the smoke rising up from the ashtray burning my eyes, I gave voice to my frustration and deep desire to leave my body and feel freedom. It was a beautifully dark poem, full of profundity for a sixteen-year-old.

I finished.

I waited for his approval, his identification.

As he took a puff from his cigarette, he looked down to the cold, concrete floor, then straight into my eyes with conviction and compassion, doing his very best to protect me from more pain. "That's great, Robbie," he said. "But don't show anyone else. It could be used against you. It's *too* deep."

Confused, I said, "Okay, Dad," and left the garage with a new sense of "I am too much. I am not enough." The smoke didn't bother me anymore.

Later on, after I was completely free of eating-disorder behaviors and learned to embody myself more, I had a conversation with my husband and our best friend, Michael. Michael was a TV star in Hollywood and one of the most hilarious people I have ever met. But there was another side of Michael; behind the celebrity was a vulnerable human being. His self-deprecating humor gave friends glimpses into his challenging childhood and mental state, the glimpses eventually forming an indelible connection to one's heart. Hanging out with him made me understand that people should not be judged by what they have achieved, but rather by who they are. No one is ever protected from the pain of life, no matter what you have or how you look.

One day in the hot Malibu sun, drinking coffee in the glare while the heat of the early morning burnt through my tank top, I had a conversation with my friend and my husband that allowed me to finally confront the lie that my size was what earned me love and respect. I was thinner than I am now and still maintaining the belief that how I looked was the basis of how much people liked me. I was arguing that if I were ten pounds heavier, those I loved would not be as fond of me. They not only balked at that statement, they were genuinely horrified by it. That got my attention. I heard them, and I also heard that my belief hurt them and discounted their character and integrity. "We love you because of you. If you were a supermodel and you were a horrible person, we wouldn't like you."

And that is the truth. Nothing more. Nothing less.

Let the Sun Illuminate the Lies

By Espra

Dieting Will Make You Thin. Umm . . . False!

Eating Disorder: "If you just use enough willpower, you can lose the weight, reach your goal, and your life will finally be good."
Truth: Dieting will make you *hungry*.

Breathing is a basic biological need. Holding your breath deprives your body of oxygen, which is necessary for survival. If it is not getting enough oxygen, your body will take over and breathe for you. Your force of will cannot control this forever. Taking a big gulp of air is not a failure of willpower. Sooner or later, it is destined to happen.

Eating is a basic biological need. Dieting deprives your body of food and nourishment, which are necessary for survival. Dieting causes physical (and psychological) deprivation and hunger. If it is not getting enough nutrition, your body will take over and eat for you. Your force of will cannot control this forever. "Breaking" a diet by eating or bingeing is not a failure of willpower. Sooner or later, it is destined to happen.

Surely, you know someone (maybe yourself) who has gone on a diet, gone off, and resumed it (or another diet) later. How many diets can you recall that have come and gone over the years? Think about it this way: If these diets made people lose weight and keep it off, why would new ones need to be dreamed up? The more diets fail, the more money people spend on diets.

More and more evidence is exposing that dieting causes binge eating and weight gain. Restricting calories or consistently spending more calories than you take in causes your metabolism to decrease, causing your body to store fat. Weight loss stops because your brilliant body holds on to precious calories needed for survival.

Some people are now realizing that diets don't work. Because people are now catching on to the farce the diet industry is adjusting by disguising diets as "lifestyle changes." Let's face it, if it involves restricting amounts and/or limiting food types, imposing rules on what you can and cannot eat—it's a diet. Dieting results in repeated weight loss followed by weight gain, which is linked to physical illnesses such as cardiovascular disease, strokes, diabetes, and decreased immune function.

And speaking of dieting, here's a sneaky eating-disorder trick: Have you ever noticed that when you're dieting, your eating disorder moves the bar on weight loss? Maybe you recognize thoughts like, *Just a little lower will be even better,* or *A little more off the thighs will get you into those quadruple zero jeans,* or *Lose just a little more and you'll feel confident enough to talk to people at parties.* Come on. See it. Catch the lies. Watch the bar moving. How long does your eating disorder stay happy with any accomplishment before it pushes you a little further?

Why Do You Really Want to Lose Weight?
Eating Disorder: "Skinny people get more respect, opportunities, and relationship options in our society. You can't deny that fat people are treated differently from skinny people."
Truth: I can promise you there are many ways to meet your goals beyond forcing your body into a mold. I believe it because I have walked beside countless individuals who have discovered ways to meet their goals independently of their body's shape and size.

Watch out: Believing that your body must be a certain way to accomplish the things that people of different shapes and sizes have accomplished is thinking you're an exception to the rule.

To be fair, there seems to be some evidence to back up, some of the time, some of the "benefits" of eating disorders that clients have taught me over the years. But you must consider the short-term benefits versus the long-term benefits. Is it worth dying just so you can talk to people at parties or get the job you seek? Is it worth dying just to keep your partner from looking at someone else? Are you absolutely certain that if your body looked the way you want it to, the things you desire would be firmly in your hands? Are you 100 percent certain there are no other variables?

You and the eating disorder are not one. You have different hopes, dreams, long-term goals, and paths to tread. Even if you believe you are one with the eating disorder because it can accomplish these things for you, it is not true. You can accomplish goals and have a life of your desire without it. Very few people start out with the intent to develop an eating disorder. It merely joins you somewhere along the path.

I hope you can pinpoint what drives your eating disorder. Okay, I get it; obviously I must not know much about eating disorders because the point is to get skinny, right? But maybe there's something more to the story. Eating disorders and/or their symptoms can provide or appear to provide benefits in the short-term.

Consider the following as just a few of the reasons why people use eating-disorder behaviors and see whether some of them apply to you. As always, don't try to force them to apply if they don't.

- To be accepted
- To feel worthwhile or loveable
- To prove you are not worthwhile or loveable
- To keep someone you love
- To be different, unique, or stand out
- To get back at someone who has hurt you
- For protection
- To be admired or to be good at something
- For self-punishment
- To be nurtured
- To help others see your emotional pain or suffering

Here are just a few of the bottom-line emotions that drive eating disorders and/or related behaviors: feeling disgusting, worthless, unlovable, invisible, alienated, flawed, or bad (due to some reason that you may or may not be able to put your finger on).

In terms of relationships, the eating disorder may convince you that it will help your relationships by making you feel more confident and outgoing, more accepted by others, more intimate or respected. There may be the hope that your eating disorder will bring distance, protection, decreased expectations, or the chance to avoid intimacy.

 What does your eating disorder convince you is obtainable by using eating-disorder behaviors, losing weight, having the perfect body, or even having the illness itself? Does it tell you that these things will be harder or impossible to accomplish without your eating disorder? Write down these expectations.

Your eating disorder may be driven by severe judgment and insults heaped on you by peers, siblings, other family members, or dating partners. Others in your life may criticize your body and reinforce your feelings of worthlessness. Dating partners are often the perpetrators of this verbal, physical, and sexual abuse. And so often, it is a secret that is hidden by shame, because the battering words are believed to be true. Increased efforts to "do better" at eating-disorder behaviors often feel like the only hope for being loved and accepted. "Who do I need to be for you to accept me?" you may ask. Like Robyn, you will find that being skinny is not the route to self-esteem and love.

The Real Payoffs of an Eating Disorder

Eating Disorder: "Don't fall for this one. You've seen the outcome; there's no way to deny it, because it's a *fact*. Others notice and want to be around thin people. Take that, you know-it-alls!"

Truth: Your eating disorder does not allow you to see beyond a short-term and immediate goal. Your longer-term goals (with which you may be out of touch or not even know) are ignored and not considered. For example, lying and deception (which may violate your long-term values) are constant companions of eating disorders. Ongoing behavior that conflicts with your values increases shame, erases self-respect, and erodes relationships.

Eating disorders (Anorexia Nervosa, Bulimia Nervosa, and Binge Eating Disorder) are serious mental illnesses. Anorexia has a high rate of suicide and has the highest mortality rate of all mental illnesses. Eating disorders often seem to develop lives of their own by overtaking the thoughts, emotions, behaviors, spirits, and identities of those they inhabit.

The eating disorder can tell you that it will ensure you have what you perceive as special and highly desirable relationships with others. But when acting out of your eating disorder, these relationships are often superficial and conditional, based on appearance, and continued out of obligation. Conflict or tension and withdrawal by loved ones are typical, though there may be increased interaction. Social and dating relationships lack depth and emotional intimacy due to preoccupation with food, your body, eating, compensating for ingested calories, and withdrawal to engage in eating-disorder behaviors.

The eating disorder fails to respect others as individuals as well. Although it is true that some people can't see beyond cheeks, thighs, and pounds, other people can. Please give people the chance to speak for themselves about what they value and like. Please give other people the respect of believing them (or at least pretending you do) when they tell you the truth about how they see you. Please do not insult me by telling me that therapists are supposed to see things this way. As I tell my clients, therapist wages don't pay me enough to be a liar.

 List three of your long-term values. Put an "x" by any that are regularly violated because of your eating disorder. The eating disorder will only take you so far if you are living out of sync with your core values. Keep this list and read it regularly to help you talk back to the eating disorder.

Keep looking at the eating disorder's lies. Consider that you and your eating disorder do not have to be one and the same. Since you are not an exception to the rest of the human race (and if you believe that people have an essence that is essentially good) then consider, too, that you might also have an authentic identity outside of your disorder.

With education, help, hope, and perseverance, you can sift through the rubble to gather and mold together pieces of the worthwhile, lovable, and true identity that is uniquely yours.

Fight the good fight.
Go against the grain.
Question your eating disorder.
Do something even when it feels too difficult.
Live.

Today, check in with yourself and question anything you feel adamant about; it could be the eating disorder. Ask yourself: does the thought you are having serve you in your new quest for recovery and self-worth? Be honest about it. If you find that the belief speaks against your well-being, throw it out. If it is one of self-worth, keep it, and know that you have just taken one more step toward victory.

6.

From the Life Raft
to the Shore

Northern Shore Beauty
and Casted Spells of Ugliness

By Robyn

Walking the evergreen streets of North Sydney always brought with it a sense of giddy anticipation mixed with a constant running motor of anxiety. My feeling of unworthiness went everywhere with me, including all the places that brought me joy. North Sydney is a place where both art and corporations mix, creating an alluring cocktail of possibilities. Settled within layers of deep history, mirrored in the old Sydney town of residential homes and ocean shores, then sprinkled with the newness of high-rises and hip establishments, the Northern Shores represented old money and new elegance. It was a place I loved to be.

I was drawn to North Sydney in my late teens. My parents had agreed to send me to a performing arts school in Sydney, and they had decided to move us from the central coast into the suburbs of Sydney in order to prevent the two-hour each way train commute that we all endured daily until the move. McDonald College of Performing Arts was a private school filled with talented wannabes who mostly came from wealthy homes. I was not one of them (from a wealthy home that is), but I pretended to be. My mother managed to get me a bursary (a partial scholarship) for the school. She was as committed to supporting my dreams as I was to following them. Melinda Williams walked into the school like she owned it. Tall, with a gymnast's physique and stunning crystal-blue eyes, Melinda was a rising childhood star. She had what we all wanted. Her own sense of importance made me want to be a part of what she was offering—her laughter (ladylike) and her presence (captivating). Melinda came from a newly broken home and lived with her father and stepmother in the suburbs of North Sydney, McMahons Point. I had passed this train stop with my mother plenty of times while traveling to and from her workplace or her lupus specialist, where I would sit in the waiting room, anxious to hear her blood count results, bringing with them either a sense of being able to breathe again or a sense of doom. But now Melinda was going to open my eyes and show me not only North Sydney, but the life that I had been waiting for, the life of an actor—glamour, spritzas (half wine, half soda water), and all the gifts that money can afford.

No one tells you that eating disorders are *ugly*. When I was enmeshed in my eating disorder, I felt the opposite. I believed it would keep me safe and in control, and make me desirable. I thought it was there to protect me from *myself*. I felt applauded and admired for my overly thin body, and snidely giggled at when I was larger. I defined myself based on how I believed I was being judged by the women around me. I walked those streets of North Sydney as both a binge eater and a near anorexic. I felt approved of when I was thin and wanted to hide or apologize for myself when I was larger than I wanted to be. However, I always felt larger than I wanted to be, even at my thinnest. This was one of the abusive ways that my eating disorder kept me in check, like a school bully with his or her fist.

I experienced a sense of coolness, even peace, when I was thin—but without absolutely *any* sense of self. Somehow, being nearly anorexic gave me a feeling of belonging and an illusion of control that made me feel acceptable. This feeling of acceptability was stamped into my psyche, as was the sense memory that measured my happiness. The problem with this was that it was rare and unpredictable. Underneath lay no foundation and no understanding of how to find and measure my sense of self. I couldn't self-soothe as I aimlessly followed the directions of the eating disorder. My body image was so entwined with my passion to be a working actor that the failure of not fitting the model of "thin, stunning, and flawless" dictated my life. I needed my eating disorder to keep me in line; it was my measuring stick for success. Dylan's abuse, too, made it easier and told me a more compelling story for why I needed to be thin. I used his abuse and aligned it with the eating disorder's, a double whammy of protection against myself. It was a painful existence and so unnecessary.

I joined my first acting agency, also in North Sydney, at the age of sixteen. It was tucked behind a high-end shopping mall in the heart of everything that was happening. I would anticipate meeting my agent and hope that my body elicited praise instead of the far more frequent sense of not being good enough. It was not uncommon for the agent's assistant to comment on my weight. I remember her telling me that I could afford to lose some pounds, as she compared me to one of my childhood friends who was also on the agency's roster. My friends were stunning with model-like attributes. I felt like an ugly duckling beside them. I also remember a photographer telling me how horrible my smile was when taking my headshots. "You mustn't smile," he said. "You'll ruin my photos!" I laughed at his antics, but came away with a new rule for myself. I took both the assistant's and photographer's statements as gospel and allowed these memories of being put in my place to remind me of how little chance I had of succeeding.

Later, Dylan and I lived on the Northern Shores as we battled it out and damaged our future together. But many wonderful things happened in North Sydney too. I created strong friendships and memories that still make my heart spill over with delight. Life is made up of both pain and joy; I understand that now. I got my first big break as an actor when I lived there, acting alongside Sam Neil, Greta Scacchi, and an amazing, established Australian cast that I felt both blessed and overwhelmed to be around. I went to my first movie premiere, too. I watched myself up on the cinema screen with my mother by my side. (My mother praised; I criticized.) After the premiere and photos, we tipsily walked home through the streets of McMahons Point with no shoes on; our feet ached from the newly purchased heels we both wore for the special celebration. My mum's feet, eroded by the side effects of lupus, had no padding to soften the impact from bone to road. Still, she giggled, grateful for the lubrication of the champagne we had shared. Nothing would get in the way of celebrating her youngest daughter's success. I had my twenty-first birthday celebration there as well. I discovered life in all its fullness there. I had my first panic attack there, and my first real heartbreak, too.

When I finally got the courage (fueled by panic attacks) to cut off my relationship with Dylan, my eating disorder began to take on other forms. I always felt like I was waiting for something horrible to happen or that I was on the verge of going crazy. I thought every feeling I had was real and that if I just stopped for even a moment, the feelings would engulf me. Taking refuge at my parents' home in Belfield, I clung onto my dad's back as he piggy-backed me around the living room, both of us screaming: "Fuck off, panic attacks! You will not get me." At twenty-two years old, both my dad and I were petrified of who I had become and feared for my sanity. Too thin, malnourished, and unable to fight off the consequences of my eating disorder, I began to suffer even more severe panic attacks. All the years of trying to be in control—of myself, of my mum's health, and of my own destiny—left me feeling emotionally robbed. I wish I could say that the end of my eating disorder was near. But it was not. It took me another seven years to say, "I'm done."

I am a sensitive soul. I see who I was as a child when I look into the eyes of my own daughter, Lilly. Her creativity, her passion to be heard, and her deep empathy for others make me brace myself at times. I take comfort in knowing that I am healthy and aware of my children's traits—some mine, some their father's, and some that they came into the world with. They have their own story that I cannot control, just as I could not control my mum's disease. But I can be here for them—healthy, present, and accepting. One day when getting out of the car after picking both girls up from school, I asked Lilly where her brand-new poncho was. "I don't know! I don't know!" she wailed, as if I had asked her where her little sister was after losing her. The panic began to rise in her, and she literally ran from me as if I were a monster. I asked her firmly but neutrally to come back to me. In an attempt to honor her feelings but to also encourage her take in her surroundings, as they were in reality, I put my arm around her shoulders and asked her to look into my eyes so she could be sure to see my truth. "Lilly, can you see that Mommy is not angry? I just asked you where you poncho was. Can you see that this is all that is going on?" She nodded with tears in her eyes.

Her emotions had already begun to consume her, like mine used to. But now I know better, and I can help her as a parent. I can teach her to self-soothe, something my parents didn't know how to do. My mum was always there to console me, but I never learned how to console myself. As I went on to tell Lilly that there was nothing else happening that brought about the need for fear, she began to understand and come to. We talked about where she'd last left the poncho, and whether it was in her classroom cubby. "But what if I can't find the poncho, Mom?" She began to panic again. "Then we will learn that when we take things off at school, we need to put them in your cubby so you know where they are. But right now you believe it is in your classroom. So tomorrow we will pick it up. It is not a big deal. Okay?" "Okay." She smiled. The following day we retrieved the poncho from where she had left it, in her classroom cubby.

I continued to lose endless days in my mid- to late twenties as I intensely focused on concocting ways to either stay thin or lose weight. I had finally lost the ability to *stay* thin for long periods of time, so most of my time was now spent on trying to get back there. My weight fluctuation wreaked havoc on my acting career. But I see now that it also became a way that I was quietly beginning to say no to the eating disorder, and establish some form of truth outside of the tiny world I had been living in with my illness. It was still there and had a presence of authority, to be sure, but its spell was beginning to wear off. I just didn't know how to break it completely. I had moments where I questioned its truth, and with it came moments of awareness that it was I who allowed my eating disorder to take me down—and that it would take my life if I let it.

Working in a corporate office as a temp, I got a much-awaited call from my agent. I lived for those calls. There was an audition that day in North Sydney for a telephone commercial. Immediately I checked in with my body, and the eating disorder shut me down. *You look fat and unsophisticated. Say no to the audition and don't waste your time. You won't get it anyway.* For a while now, I had been growing sick and tired of being dictated to by this feeling of unworthiness. I had begun to recognize what was happening in my relationship with the eating disorder, as I had during my relationship with Dylan. I knew that just because both of them provided a ton of noise when I went against their directions, I still had the choice to change things and say no. That day, as I sat at the reception desk filtering calls for a bunch of fun-loving, money-hungry traders, I began to question myself:

Is it true that the casting agency wants only wafer-thin glamour girls for the role they are casting? No.

Is it true that they will immediately judge me for what I look like and not for how I act? No.

Is it indeed true that I am fat? No.

The eating disorder wanted to jump in, but with every question I asked myself, I abruptly cut off its voice. I had become willing to wait and let the facts reveal themselves instead of beating myself up with lies. I decided to go to the audition and own all that I was. Even if it was just for the duration of the audition, I promised myself to have confidence and not allow the eating disorder to come into the audition room with me. It would stay in the waiting room with all the other gorgeous young ladies, comparing my thighs with theirs. But I walked into the audition room alone, unapologetic, and was hired later that day.

To this day questioning the truth and the story I tell myself is a source of empowerment. I see this same sense of empowerment come naturally to my daughter Chloe. Instinctively, she often pauses without a word and observes the world around her. Sometimes when I tell her she can't do something, she will begin to whine, then stop and say, "But why, Mommy?" Chloe symbolizes normality—whatever that is. She almost seems foreign to me. With a glorious sense of humor and an innate sense of self, she doesn't appear to have that invisible barrier of fear that Lilly, Tim, and I share. One day at our little town fair, I put both Lilly and Chloe on a kids' ride that spun around. Lilly was thrilled as the ride began to twirl slowly, though quite quickly for a toddler. She lifted her hands with pure excitement and reckless abandon, while Chloe looked over to me with a look in her eyes that said, "How the hell did I get here, and who are you people?" I laughed with a joy that will forever remain with me. She is our teacher, and we are hers, providing lessons of balance, creativity, the unforgiving power of fear, and the true sense of self that can combat that. What a beautiful life. God is good.

The Beauty and the Beast Within

By Espra

Emotions 101

Eating Disorder: "Skip this section. Jump to the important part. You already know everything you need to know about emotions. The faster you get rid of the bad ones, the better off you are."

Truth: A lack of understanding about emotions and how they work is an obstacle to recovery. Learning how emotions operate will give you an edge in managing your feelings, thoughts, and behaviors, without needing an eating disorder to do so for you.

One of the most important things to understand about emotions is that they are physically based. Every emotion is created in hardwired circuits deep in our brain. These circuits activate physical responses to incoming information before we are even consciously aware of what is going on. Our brain has a core system that constantly scans for information coming into our awareness from what we see, hear, taste, touch, or smell. When your brain detects incoming information it automatically searches its existing database for your experiences and beliefs about yourself, others, and the world. When your brain locates what it *perceives* to be a match in its database, it deposits the information there. Then your brain instantly sets off a pre-organized pattern of physical changes in your body. Each set of physical changes has been fine-tuned over thousands of years to get your body to do what is needed for you to have the best chance of survival and well-being. These body sensations and changes are what we call emotions.

We naturally refer to emotions in terms of their physical characteristics when we say things like, "I was so ashamed I wanted to crawl under a rock and hide," or "I was frozen with fear." Robyn describes waiting to see if her mom's test results would decrease Robyn's fear so she could "breathe again." The brain decides which chemicals and impulses to send through the body to get the body to either slow down or deliver additional energy. Emotional responses are instant and instinctive. The brain's ability to put our bodies into action works with a physiological efficiency that is more like passing, rather than dribbling, to move a basketball down a court. It is essential to our survival.

As an emotion surges through the body, creating its unique pattern of physical effects, it hijacks our attention and takes our thoughts with it. The emotion dictates our thoughts and then our thoughts fuel the emotion to keep it going. This is what's happening when we say something like, "I was so angry I couldn't think straight." Our brains begin to collect thoughts that increase the emotion. For example, feeling embarrassed and ashamed causes us to think about things we don't like about ourselves and our failures. Our survival has relied on emotions and thoughts fueling each other. If you were backed into a corner by a cougar, fear might get your body to try to fight or scare the cougar away. Your survival would depend on your thoughts reminding you of how afraid you are, while thoughts about the cougar's pretty coat would decrease your brain's production of physical energy and probably get you killed. There are other times when our brains register information that leads to emotions that set off a chain of thoughts and behaviors that is harmful instead of helpful. For example, if a police officer backs you into a corner and your brain plugs the information into a threat database, like with the cougar, your body might instinctively try to scare the officer away. That response would be anything but a helpful course of action.

Since emotions are biological responses that affect the entire body, trying to push away painful emotions is like trying to push water. You can expend precious energy until it is depleted as you work to slow, stop, or speed up emotions' flow. Attempts to push emotions down or make them move faster only increases their pressure and energy, as well as your misery. This approach does not level out emotions at all. You need a new approach to emotions to stabilize the chaos you might experience in their wake. Instead of trying to change the course of your emotions, consider learning how to allow the constant current of your emotions to work in your favor in the way they were created to work. Emotions are messengers that can bring information to us (and others) about what is going on around us and ways we can respond. If we know how to use them, emotions give us an advantage and help us respond to life in an informed and meaningful way.

Think about the brain like a sonar (the underwater relative of the radar) in a submarine, which is used to provide information for navigation, communication, and detection of objects. Always on alert, like your brain, the sonar constantly scans for information about what is in the surrounding area. A submarine crew diligently monitors its sonar and carefully assesses incoming information. It remains ready to engage immediately in a well-rehearsed, efficient pattern of actions when necessary. When picked up by the sonar, battleships, submarines, whales, and oceanic mountains each have unique characteristics that indicate to the crew which course of action is needed. The course of action is chosen based on what the evidence suggests would be most likely to keep the submarine and its crew alive and unharmed. In your brain this same process occurs automatically, without conscious intervention. This is why emotions can be hard to change.

What I'm talking about is paying attention to the signals as information and carefully observing your sensations, thoughts, urges, posture, and behaviors. When did the first signals start? Exactly what incoming information did your brain react to? Name these things. Only after clearly identifying and allowing all of the information into your awareness can you deliberately consider accurate responses to the original data that your brain picked up. In this place of information you become able to use your brain to override the reactions that are being dictated by your body. From this place it becomes possible to respond deliberately and decide what step to take first or next. Many who have used eating-disorder behaviors to cope with emotions find that they can begin to see a first, best step, which is different than eating, restricting, or getting rid of calories to cope with emotion.

I use the sonar metaphor below as a way to help my clients understand and work with emotions and reactions. If a submarine crew does not carefully read the incoming data on the sonar screen, they may create a disaster by firing a torpedo at a whale or oceanic mountain. The same is true for how we must respond to events in our lives.

SONAR

Signals from your body that your brain has picked up incoming information.

Observe, don't ignore both the signals and incoming information.

Name your body reactions and thoughts.

Allow the incoming information, your signals, and your stories to flow.

Respond deliberately to the situation, without reacting to your stories about it.

Learn how to use your SONAR.

1. **Pay attention to signals from your body for a day, watching for a physical response to show up.** Start with a small response to an event, if you can catch one.

2. **Observe the signals and incoming information.** Examples of incoming information: My family member poured water out of a pot and then told me I was supposed to pour the water out twenty minutes ago. Then I heard him or her sigh.

3. **Name your body reactions and thoughts about the incoming information.** My body reactions: My forehead tensed and my brows wrinkled together. It hurt my forehead a little. My thoughts: I messed up again. I do everything wrong. I mess up everything, like

losing at badminton yesterday. My family member is sick of being around a fat, slow idiot who can't do anything right. Nobody wants a stupid mess-up around. I wish I could just disappear.

4. **Allow the incoming information, your signals, and your stories to flow.** Incoming information: I saw one action, heard one sentence, and heard a sigh. Signals: Right away my head scrunched until it started to hurt. Story: Look how fast my mind added that I'm a fat, slow, idiot who needs to disappear . . . all from one action, a sentence, and a sigh! I'm really good at creating stories. (We all are.)

5. **Respond to the situation.** I say, "I thought I'd read the directions carefully. I'll read them again to see if I need to do it differently next time." Action: I will stay right here instead of letting my stories send me out of the room.

• •

Use your sonar to guide you in responding to life events. In the above example, if the family member threw the pot at you, disappearing might have been the best thing to do. Use only what is actually showing up to gather the information you need. It is from this place that you can respond to information and life with more wisdom, awareness, intention, and power than when your chemistry and body dictate your thinking and behavior. This is authentic power and authentic power is a building block of recovery.

Allowing emotions to work in their natural way helps to keep them from getting stuck or dammed up and gives us protection against "drowning in emotion." Working with our emotions helps decrease the unnecessary suffering they can cause by sweeping away our thoughts, hijacking our ability to think clearly, and dragging our behaviors along with them. Working with, instead of against, emotions is essential if you want full recovery that heals not only eating-disorder behaviors, but also eating-disorder urges and thoughts. Over time, working with the inherent way that emotions flow increases your ability to respond deliberately to life in the most effective ways possible and contributes to a life that feels worth living.

Know What's Eating You

Eating Disorder: "No brainer. Being *fat* is eating you."

Truth: Early in treatment when I ask my clients how they feel, they will usually reply, "I feel fat." You may feel fat, but notice how you feel fatter when you feel bad about things other than your body.

Most people can identify only about four to six emotions. Once you learn how to label emotions, how they function, and how they are expressed verbally and nonverbally, you can see them at work across species. (I know when my dog experiences happiness, love, disgust, anger, and shame because he shows the same posture and gestures that humans show with similar emotions.) People tend to cope better with hard emotions after learning more about their nature.

Looking at emotions in their most basic form can help decrease your hard feelings about having hard feelings. My clients often find it helpful to look at the benefits of emotions through the example of being a member of a tribe with the need to protect and help one another survive: You head to a field of planted crops and see a herd of animals grazing on the food that you planted to help your tribe survive the winter. Your eyes quickly take in this situation and your thoughts immediately conclude that the food you need for survival is about to be lost. Your body instantly creates physical and mental energy as a resource and sends chemicals, signals, and impulses that prepare your body to fight or chase away the grazers in order to keep your food. We call this physical energy anger, and in this example anger would increase your chance of survival.

The emotion of fear helps us avoid danger as it either energizes or shuts down the body to get the threat away from us (fight), get us away from the threat (flee), or hide (freeze). The brain searches its database, quickly determines which fear response to create in our bodies, and makes it happen. Sometimes the automatic reaction urges us to do what is most effective under the circumstances, and other times it does not. When we are afraid or anxious, our breathing gets shallow and quick, muscles tense, and the heart races. Once fear is surging chemically through the body and the brain, it brings our thoughts along, using them as fuel to continue to propel the emotion. However, if fear is driving your body to run away when you need to interact in a scary social situation, it will not help you survive, and it will get in your way. With fear, sometimes if you need to act, you cannot; and sometimes if you need to mellow out, you cannot. It is hardly possible to engage in action that is logical because the body and the brain dictate both current thinking and continue to bring thoughts along for the ride.

The emotion of sadness pulls our attention inward while we regroup after a loss or disappointment. Ideally it lets others know that we need support, protection, and closeness. When sadness flows through us unobstructed, it helps us gather time and support as we grieve, and gather our reserves to resume our lives in a changed way. When sadness cannot flow through us naturally, it can lead to long-term withdrawal, avoidance, and depression.

Embarrassment and guilt act like glue for relationships as they help us refrain from doing things that compromise our relationships with others and ourselves. These emotions get us to mend any damage we have done in relationships. For example, embarrassment and guilt can keep us from lying or stealing, or help us repair the damage to ourselves and others when we do. However, when guilt persists after we have mended the harm we caused, it can become destructive. Guilt and embarrassment (or shame) can become like playground bullies that jump out at us, beat us up, and knock us down over and over, just because they can. In this way, misplaced guilt and shame can take our freedom and drain our spirit. If you consistently feel guilt because of what, when, or how much you have eaten, this guilt can take over your thoughts, your behaviors, and your life. Robyn exposes the risks of misplaced shame when she talks about feeling approved of when she was thin and wanting to hide or apologize when her body was larger than she wanted it to be. This is an example of how eating-disorder behaviors like bingeing, restricting, or purging seem to relieve guilt and shame. The instant relief encourages the behaviors to be repeated. The emotions feel like the beast within, and the eating disorder that seems to tame the beast can kill you.

Jealousy and envy give us energy so we can improve ourselves, our environment, and hold on to what's important to us. The emotion of envy is evident when young siblings propel their development forward as they compete to outdo one another. But sometimes these emotions can lead to behaviors that alienate others and get in the way of improving ourselves or our environment. If envy or jealousy motivates you to strive at any cost to be "skinnier," "restrict better," or get rid of ingested calories to fit an ideal or to be better than others, it can destroy your relationships, your health, and it can take your life.

In order to survive we must avoid things that can physically, emotionally, or mentally harm us. When we say another's actions "turn my stomach," or that rotten potatoes make me "turn up my nose," it is the emotion of disgust motivating our body to turn away from what might harm us. It is horrific and damaging when individuals feel disgust during contact with things or people who are causing them harm, yet still have to depend on that environment for their survival or well-being. If you are in a situation like this, seek help from a safe and trusted individual. Too often people with eating disorders feel disgust with themselves or their bodies. If such disgust drives you to turn away from yourself, mentally beat yourself up, harm yourself, or want to destroy or kill yourself, your disgust is leading you into, instead of away from, danger. Please get help.

Pride serves us well when it energizes and motivates us to build on our accomplishments. Eating disorders abuse pride, as they create a sense of identity and uniqueness in "being the best" at using eating-disorder behaviors. Pride destroys people when they strive to do something better or be admired for things that cause harm to themselves or others. It is particularly harmful when emotions like love or happiness careen into emotions like shame, guilt, and anger. It is common for people with eating disorders to feel, for example, a spark of happiness, then immediately have the thought that they don't deserve or are not worthy to feel happy. This leads to feeling ashamed for feeling happy. This happens and you need to be on the lookout for it, catch it, and treat it because it will get in the way of recovery.

Your belief about hard emotions might be that they will drown and destroy you unless you find a way to stop them, speed them along, or push them down. Many of my clients speak of the benefits of eating, bingeing, purging, or restricting nutrition to control emotions. However, those benefits are short-lived so the behaviors are often used over and over again.

Since emotions are biological, being aware of our physical sensations is often our first clue that an emotion has shown up. We can also notice our thoughts, urges, statements, body language, and behaviors to understand what is happening emotionally. Once you notice the signals that an emotion is present, carefully observe all incoming information. Then name everything you observe about the emotion. (Just labeling an emotion can sometimes decrease its intensity.) Since emotions neither go away nor remain at the most extreme intensity forever, the goal is to focus on changes in their intensity and to let the emotions settle down to a point where you can think about what is going on. Thinking about an emotion doesn't mean that you try to stop it, understand what's wrong with you for having the emotion, or decry how weak you are or how you "should" feel instead.

Know What's Running the Show

Eating Disorder: "One thing you can trust is that people lie to you. Not many people are honest enough to tell you that you are disgusting to them."

Truth: Most of us have times when we think we know what someone is thinking about us. Most of us have times when we think others are judging our appearance. It is possible to know for sure what you think, believe, or intend; but, despite convincing thoughts to the contrary, it is impossible to know for certain what others think, believe, or intend.

Most people who struggle with eating disorders can become consumed with thinking they know what others are thinking about them, and it is mostly negative. My clients frequently inform me about negative thoughts I have about them when I don't even know I'm having those thoughts. Can you see the error here? It seems that mind reading and personalizing often come first and can play a part in causing an eating disorder. Once the eating disorder enters the scene, this sort of mind reading gets a turbo boost, and the cycle takes on a life of its own.

To put this information about emotions into a coherent package, consider this example: An emotion typically starts when something happens. The event can be internal, like a thought about the future or a memory of the past. Or an emotion can be prompted by an external event, like getting passed over for a job. For example, my clients rattle off such automatic thoughts as, "I'm fat. Fat people don't get good jobs." "I don't deserve it anyway." "I'm a failure." "I'm stupid, fat, worthless, and ugly." "There's nothing about me that stands out." The list goes on and on. Do you recognize any of these thoughts as your own? If so, does it surprise you that these thoughts are more related to eating-disorder thinking than unique to you? Interpretations about being defective come from shame and create more shame. Shame pushes us to hide (avoid future auditions) or conform to be more desirable (get "skinny enough" in order to succeed). The eating disorder is firmly in control as dieting or compensating for calories becomes the path to accomplishing the goal, or bingeing or restricting is used to temporarily soothe the pain. This is how thoughts, urges, and behaviors can be dictated by ignored or overwhelming emotions.

Therefore, it is important for us to know when our emotions are running the show. It makes sense to have particular emotions in certain circumstances. However, just because you have an emotion doesn't mean that it is motivating your thoughts or behaviors to do what is helpful to you in the situation. Step back, look at the facts, and challenge the eating-disorder thoughts for yourself.

A thought is a thought. A flower is a flower. A feeling is a feeling. What you see with your eyes is what you see. An opinion about any of those things is merely an opinion about that thing. Just because you happen to have a thought, a feeling, an opinion, or a belief about something does not mean it is necessarily accurate. If you can see it, hear it, taste it, touch it, or smell it, you can be sure it's accurate because information from the world around you confirms it. For example, there is a difference between someone's eyebrows wrinkling together (which you can see) and that person being mad at you (a story your mind might create about the wrinkled brow). Some people wrinkle their brow when they have a headache or are concentrating. Like Robyn, your recovery depends on breaking free from thinking that every feeling you have is relevant and factual. Your recovery journey depends, in part, on gradually exposing yourself to feelings in these ways in order to eventually trust that the hard feelings won't engulf you.

Robyn always felt larger than she wanted to be, "fat," even at her thinnest. Therapists who specialize in working with eating disorder recovery have interventions that can help you check the accuracy of your own thoughts, beliefs, or perceptions about your body. Until then, the eating disorder can tell you whatever it decides, and you are at risk of thinking, "Oh, yes, you're right," when it is actually selling you poison and you are drinking it, no questions asked.

As you are going about your life, pay attention for just one hour. Notice when you add a thought or create a story in your mind about what is happening or why it is occurring. Use a pen and paper, your phone (there are apps for counting), or any sort of counter. Anytime you have a thought that goes beyond what you can directly see, hear, taste, touch, or smell, that thought is an addition to or a story about the information that is going into your brain. You are then observing your story instead of the information that your brain initially detected. Count how many stories your mind creates during the course of that hour. Try not to beat yourself up when you notice more stories than information because that's the way our brains work. The purpose of this tool is to help you learn to notice the difference between incoming information and the stories your brain adds to that information.

Example: If you are in the mall and thinking that others are disgusted and think you are fat when they look at you, pause. Carefully observe how many people you actually see looking at you and how many people's eyes move up and down or become fixed on your body. Many of my clients begin to learn that very few people even look at others, much less stare beyond a quick glance. Despite being convinced that you know the thoughts of other people, you cannot. You might need to keep track of how many people look at you versus how many don't. You need to have a count in order to factually determine whether it is 10, 50, 80, or 100 percent of others. Otherwise, you are making up things in your mind about what is going on, and eating disorders thrive on the stories.

• •

Even if you choose to listen to your eating disorder and believe it about certain things, please don't let it insult your intelligence by falling for those things that could be proven false if you just took some time to carefully observe the incoming information. Then name the stories your thoughts are creating about what you observe. Once you practice and get the hang of this skill, you—like Robyn passing on her hard-earned wisdom to Lilly—can also teach others to identify incoming information more accurately. Imagine what true power could manifest if mothers, fathers, families, friends, loved ones, and society could learn and pass on the skill of taking in the signals, then deliberately observing and naming them as a way to help themselves and others decrease and cope with painful emotions. Even if, just once, a painful emotion could be changed by exposing its misfiring, it is worth the time and effort.

Get into Your Right Mind
Eating Disorder: "They are saying you need to do a better job at controlling your feelings. That's why I'm here for you. Now they're saying that I lie to you. You can't trust anything they say."
Truth: Eating disorders are often about pushing feelings away, pushing them down, or giving them an outlet. We are not encouraging you to manage your feelings in any of these ways.

Trying to pull away from an eating disorder is like jumping from a sinking ship onto a life raft. Rather than drifting, let's look at how to move your life raft in a direction that you ultimately choose to go. Learning to juggle awareness of your emotions so you can respond deliberately instead of automatically reacting can work like paddles on a boat. It helps you go from fighting the current and drifting helplessly at the mercy of your emotions to navigating the rapids and obstacles in the direction you desire.

Historically, people were often encouraged in therapy to change their thoughts in order to change their emotions. This approach can be helpful. A problem with this approach for many of my clients is that people with a predisposition for emotional sensitivity, perfectionistic thinking, and putting themselves down wonder what's wrong with them when they can't just change their thoughts to get rid of an emotion. We now know about different ways to shift emotions, especially through our actions. Trying to think differently in order to change painful emotions can be like trying not to think about the painful burning sensation in your hand after it gets burned. Acting differently is like putting ice on your hand to ease the pain, which helps you think about it less while you perform the first aid necessary to minimize the damage. Our minds and bodies tend to respond more quickly with emotional change when we first change our *actions* than when we try to change our *thoughts*. Once our actions begin to shift our emotions, it is less difficult to change our thoughts.

When Robyn had the urge to avoid auditions because she felt too fat, she knew the emotion of shame was working against her. Her shame, gone unchecked, might have pushed her to restrict, purge, or avoid auditions until she was "skinny enough"—or all three. Robyn saw the signals, and then observed her body, thoughts, and emotions and what they were urging her to do. She named what she was observing. Then she allowed all of the information to flow through her as she sorted the actual data from her stories about the data. If an emotion is consuming you and getting you to think and do things that are not helpful under the circumstances, you might need to just do something different. After observing and naming what she saw and heard as well as her resulting thoughts, Robyn could evaluate whether or not it was 100 percent guaranteed that her body was getting in the way of her getting every part. She realized that, instead, it was 100 percent guaranteed that her embarrassment and disgust for her body were the factors that stood between her and getting a part, as long as they kept her from even going to auditions. She knew that the only way to get a part, which was her goal, was to go to auditions anyway. Robyn began to suspect that waiting until she was "skinny enough" (based on the eating disorder's standards) to land a part would leave her hiding and avoiding auditions forever. What disastrous outcomes this would have caused for an actress! Leaving her eating-disorder behavior at the door, Robyn took her determined, shame-filled body to the audition and immersed herself in her audition as if her life depended on it. The life Robyn dreamed of *did* depend on it.

Using her deliberately chosen response instead of her automatic reaction worked at a time when letting shame dictate her actions would only have gotten in the way. Robyn got the part. It confirmed that the emotion and the stories in her head weren't helpful (or accurate) after all. This is how Robyn's *action* of going to auditions even when she felt ashamed of her body helped lay the foundation for her recovery.

Carefully observing the signals of what is coming in and how your body and mind are responding can help you isolate responses that are more likely to be accurate. Name what you can see, hear, taste, touch, and smell. Allow the flow of incoming information as well as your conclusions about the information. Allow yourself to consider whether or not the evidence supports the accuracy of your conclusion. Then it is possible to determine an accurate course of action and respond deliberately. It is important to be aware that the issue here is more about whether or not the emotion is motivating you to do something helpful than whether or not you *like* the emotion.

For fear that I am making this sound too easy, let me assure you that it is anything but easy, and it takes a lifetime of practice for all of us. It is worth the effort, as the benefits of working *with* instead of against our emotions are life-changing.

The benefits of working *with* instead of against our emotions are life-changing.

When you observe the signals, name them, and accept them, you might find they are pushing you to do what is helpful in a particular situation. It is best to harness and use their energy and influence to your advantage. Robyn knew that her anger at her eating disorder (for continuing its efforts to convince her that her value and worth were based on the size and shape of her body) was helpful. She used her anger to help her find the energy to develop a plan for what she would do differently when her eating disorder went after her with its emotional club. Once you know what your body and mind are automatically reacting to, you can use the information to develop a plan for a new pattern of responses in the future.

A plan of action can be developed for any pattern or reaction that is predictable. This can help you override your initial urge in favor of a more useful response when one is needed. Because Robyn's pattern was so predictable, it was preventable. As Robyn put her plan into action, it focused her anger in a single direction, to uncover her worth in ways more in line with her actual goals and values. That's when she began to see her anger overpowering the last of the emotional hold that the eating disorder had on her. It was Robyn's willingness to work *with* her anger that pried the last remaining tentacles of her eating disorder from around her heart and finally freed her from its grasp.

What *Really* Protects You?

Eating Disorder: "Duh, that's easy. Me, of course! I'm the only one who really has your back. I protect you."

Truth: There are ways to protect yourself, to keep situations from hitting you as hard emotionally *and* to cope with difficult emotions once they hit. Those ways have nothing to do with the illusions and quick fixes your eating disorder uses to "protect" you from emotions.

Hopefully you are beginning to see that emotions often happen before we have the chance to influence them. However, there are things you can do to decrease the impact that difficult emotions have on you. Since your emotions are so closely related to the state of your brain and your body, looking after your body can help you decrease hard emotions and respond deliberately to them. Stabilize your nutrition using your dietician and structured eating plan as resources, rather than the eating disorder.

Physical pain, illness, and health issues, including vision and dental problems, can all make emotions harder to manage. Prescription or over-the-counter medications, herbs, or supplements (for sleep, colds, allergies, or dieting; caffeine pills; laxatives, etc.), even when taken as directed can negatively affect your emotions. Use these only as prescribed or as directed on the label. Legal as well as illicit mood-altering substances wreak havoc on emotions.

One alcoholic beverage makes it harder to see the signals, accurately assess information, and respond deliberately. I am not preaching against drinking alcohol; I am encouraging you to avoid it when you need to figure out how to respond deliberately to emotional situations. Get as much sleep as you need and no more than necessary. Sleep medications, though sometimes necessary, create low-quality sleep. If you are willing to work at it, there are many ways to promote the kind of sleep that is most beneficial. Look into those, with professional help if needed, and experiment to see if they are helpful to you. With either too much or too little sleep it's harder to see the signals, accurately assess information, and respond deliberately. Physical activities within the guidelines set by your physician and nutritionist can improve mood. Too much or a lack of physical activity is also hard on your emotions. It is all about balance.

With either too much or too little sleep it's harder to see the signals, accurately assess information, and respond deliberately.

Challenge yourself but make sure you see and take in your accomplishments. (Dieting, weight loss, and the like don't count!) Doing big and small things you enjoy while paying attention to what you're doing—and your mood while you are doing it—is important. Remember or consider your goals, values, and priorities, aside from anything related to food or your body, and let those guide your actions. These are the things that also help you build a foundation and understanding of how to find and strengthen your sense of self. If you are out of balance (deprived or in excess) in any of these areas, it could explain why you are having more difficulty with emotions at a particular time, and balancing where you can is helpful.

Remember, too, that we are talking about freedom of emotion, not freedom from emotion. It will take time for your brain to learn that emotions are not your enemy. So take a deep breath, slow down, open your eyes, involve yourself in your life, and balance your life.

Can you hear the calling?
It is the calling of purpose.
We all have it. We all can live it.
Shhh . . . listen.
Make a change.

*Today, I will take time to remind myself of the gifts
I was brought into the world with. If I don't know,
I will allow myself to think of something positive
about myself, pushing through the noise of my
eating disorder until I find it. I will then put those
gifts out into the universe where they belong and be
willing to utilize them when the invitation arises. If
my eating disorder says no, I will ask, "Why not?"—
reminding myself that it is I who has the choice.*

7.

Gather the Troops

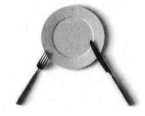

Spanish Pay Phones and Glaswegian Nightclubs

By Robyn

I love to act. Ever since I can remember, acting was what it was all about for me. At age two, I often made my mum and neighbor sit through my incoherent improvisations, full of mumbling, but also undeniable commitment. When I was a teenager, I would often spend my lunchtime writing my own scripts and then perform them in class. It was my passion, and it sprang from a deep, tangible desire to move people.

When I was nineteen, a Tony Award-winning British director came to Sydney, Australia to watch a small co-op play that his friend had directed. I happened to be in it. I was raw, but ready. The director decided he wanted me to be in his film, and just like that, it was the start to that dream I believed in back when I was all of two. At twenty-four, I had a series on TV, and by twenty-six, after much persuasion from friends who had already gone before me, I headed to where I believed big dreams could come true: Hollywood. But by then, my illness had taken over, and no matter what extraordinary opportunities came to me—and I was blessed with many "once in a lifetime" opportunities—they never were more important than my eating disorder. *When I get thin enough, I will concentrate on my career. When I get thin enough, I'll show the world who I really am.* And just like that, my dreams were eaten up by my illness that was ever so hungry for destruction.

Although I was never able to see the gifts in my life due to the wall of my illness, I always had people who believed in me and wanted to love me, if only I would let them. I believed that if I opened up, people would see my insides—the confusion, the fear, and a story that would have them judging me and running for the hills. I worked my whole life to create a persona that disguised my truth. It was the acting gig of my life!

I made decisions based on how I felt. Unfortunately, most of the time I felt unworthy and "less than." I told my new manager (who had been sending casting agents chocolates and flowers just to goad them into seeing this new Aussie actor) that I would return in six months to pick up on the opportunities he had created for me. I didn't return for five years. Needless to say, the opportunities were gone.

Within those five years, still running from my truth, I traveled back to Australia, then London and Spain, and landed in Scotland. Seeking perfection in whatever I did, I'd made a decision to study at a highly regarded Scottish music and drama academy to perfect my acting technique—but honestly, I did it to buy me time. I ran to seven countries in five years, and my eating disorder ran with me.

In the middle of the night on the dark, hauntingly quiet streets of Valencia, Spain, where I had taken a position in children's theatre as a way to run away from myself again, it wasn't uncommon for me to howl into a pay phone, sobbing to my mother, whom I had woken from her sleep. "I can't do this anymore. I can't live like this." She knew I was desperate and trapped in my illness. She was powerless (this illness is a heartbreaking experience for parents and loved ones); we both felt powerless. I had been bingeing and purging my way through Spain, spending six hours a day in the bathroom. I was unable to stop, unable to embrace anything outside of my illness. I think my mum was okay with getting the middle-of-the-night calls because she believed that the alternative (not getting them) would mean the death of her child.

In Spain, it was not uncommon to perform two to three shows a day, eating out for all meals. One day our driver was running late and our lunch break was cut short as we piggybacked shows. I had consumed the menu of the day and a carafe of cheap red wine in order to aid my purge. But to my dismay, I did not have time to purge, so upon returning to the theatre, I placed a bucket that I'd found in the bathroom behind the stage, so that when I returned after each scene, I could purge. I would run on stage as Blue-Hat Betty, with my bulging waist and bloated face, then run backstage and purge as Robbed-of-All-Dignity Robyn. Yet to many, it appeared I was living the dream.

I had learned how to cope by trying to get whatever I could to ease my discomfort in that very moment. Looking back, I am ashamed to say that, in truth, I got my mum to pay an international fee of $30,000 from her home savings so that I could be encouraged to go on living. I told her that attending the Music and Drama Academy would provide something worth living for. I *believed* this. I felt like an imposter, a fraud. I thought, and insisted to my mum, that getting the proper education, instead of passing over it due to my qualifying experience, would make me feel legitimate. I was convinced that this move would bring me some relief from the eating disorder's accusations that I was merely a fraud who deserved nothing. I insisted this would lessen my misery at the hands of the eating disorder. She prayed it would free me from the depths of my agony, and in turn bring her some freedom from her darkest fears of completely losing her daughter. I could have waited a year and paid a sixth of this fee, as I would then have been classified as a resident of the United Kingdom. But I couldn't wait; I wouldn't wait. I needed something to focus on and to bring me hope, something to project my fantasies upon. All my weary mum could see was a stranger who had the facial features (despite the swollen, ripped blood vessels in my eyes) of the child she loved so dearly and profoundly. She had long ago lost the child she raised, but she so desperately wanted her back. And like most parents, she was willing to go to any lengths—and any cost—to make that happen. If I could take back the pain I caused my mum, dear God, I would. But these are now my scars of my battle, the guilt and shame that I carry. I will move forward anyway . . . and I know this is what my mum would want.

The more I isolated myself, the more my illness grabbed hold. I would never be perfect. Life would never be perfect. To expose the lie of perfection, I needed to expose my illness that was pushing the lie. To expose my illness, I had to expose my true self.

The powerful stigma of an eating disorder (a mental illness) is always just under the surface. I had an ugly secret that, if uncovered, would reveal my vulnerability for the entire world to see. But it was this very thing that would open me to the life I had been seeking through my running. That vulnerability is now my strength. Acceptance in knowing that I could no longer do it alone was the key that unshackled me from the burden of my ugly secret. It was true that I could never do it alone, and nothing I did could change that. It came down to sharing my story and asking for help . . . or dying.

After midnight, as I lay defeated in my bed in the heart of Glasgow, Scotland, I listened to the raucous sound of two drunken Glaswegian men declaring their strength as they threw punches at each other just outside my window. It wasn't unusual for this type of scene to be the soundtrack to my weekend. I lived across from a popular nightclub that would start gathering steam in the wee hours of the morning. I would usually drown out the racket with earplugs, which were scattered around the narrow room covered in rich, purple wallpaper that hid me from the eyes of others and aided my ability to binge in secret. But on that chilly night, I decided to forgo the earplugs so the sound of the nightclub would shield me from the noise inside my head. Somehow the pounding of fists and the men's loyal friends egging them on seemed more pleasant to me than my own thoughts. I'd been drinking, and only moments before I'd been weeping on the pages of the phonebook, which was open to reveal the number of the suicide hotline. I lay on the floor, unable to balance myself when standing, and slid my hand to the phone that sat on the black, crumb-sprinkled carpet, as if it were waiting for me. But instead of calling the hotline, I called a friend from the support group I had attended a week before out of desperate need to find a solution to this horrid illness. The support group had provided me with a phone list that I would normally have thrown out after it had remained wrinkled in my handbag for weeks, collecting the crumbs from each of my binges. But that night in Glasgow, I chose to share my story with a person with whom I identified. I felt safe with her because I had witnessed her openly sharing her own story with a group that supported recovery and honored truth, and it gave me the courage to do the same.

I chose to start telling my truth to those who identified with me and wanted to help me, and in whom I trusted. This act changed my life forever.

Calling for Backup

By Espra

Eating Disorder: "You don't need anyone. Are you kidding me? If you tell people about this, they will think you are crazy and you will surely be taken to the nuthouse."
Truth: You cannot do this alone.

Your eating disorder takes a harsh toll on your relationships. Still, gathering a strong support network to fight your eating disorder is critical. Here we've outlined the things that are important to consider and to ask of others when you are working to create a necessary safety net for your survival and for your recovery.

Medical Care

Tell your medical provider the truth about your eating disorder and symptoms. Your urge will be to downplay the severity and frequency of your behaviors and symptoms. Don't. It will keep you from recovery. Find a physician who can assess, as well as help you monitor and manage your physical health and medical needs. Start by having a thorough medical assessment by a provider who is familiar with the many medical risks associated with eating disorders as soon as possible. If your physician is willing but needs additional information about medical evaluation and management of eating disorders, direct him or her to the Academy of Eating Disorders (AED) website's educational report on recognizing and managing the medical risks for individuals with eating disorders that is available for reading or to download. The American Medical Association (AMA) website also has an educational video on screening and managing eating disorders that was developed in conjunction with the National Eating Disorder Association (NEDA) and AED.

Ask your physician about the laboratory, cardiac, and other tests that are necessary to evaluate and treat patients with eating disorders. You will need to discuss medical risks, contraindications, and recommendations for all medications and over-the-counter substances you are using, exercise (frequency, intensity, and duration), and other considerations.

Make sure your physician does not focus exclusively on body mass index or weight to diagnose the severity of your eating disorder and to determine appropriate medical interventions. Make sure that the focus of stabilizing your eating disorder does not include a weight-loss plan. Ask your physician if he or she is willing to coordinate your care with your other providers. Make a plan for the frequency and types of measures that will be needed in order to monitor your medical status. If your physician is willing and able to take this approach to assessing and helping you manage your eating disorder, you are well on your way.

 Write down all your symptoms and eating-disorder behaviors. Then look over your list and honestly evaluate it for accuracy. Identify what you have left out or minimized and correct it now. Take a deep breath and take this list with you to your physician's visit. Be sure to give the list to your physician.

• •

Faith and Finding a Power Greater Than Ourselves

Some say that living in the throes of an eating disorder is a spiritual crisis. It can rob your spirit, your essence, and it can compromise your long-term values. In turn, your self-esteem and self-worth sink lower. A twelve-step group like Eating Disorders Anonymous (among others) can help you live a life outside of obsession. Many of these organizations talk about a "higher power." Use language that works for you, rather than choosing to go to or avoid groups based on how this reference is made. People use the phrase "higher power" to refer to a wide range of strengths that individuals strive to tap into in the process of healing. People may or may not relate "higher power" to deities with whom they identify (God, Jesus, Allah, Universe, etc.). Seek your own source of strength and use it, while you accept others as they do the same. Take what works for you and leave the rest.

Other Support Groups

A local eating-disorder facility or one of your healthcare providers may be able to give you referrals for support groups in your area. Weight-loss groups are *not* what you need. Therapy groups that target identity development, assertiveness training, and general quality-of-life skills can be helpful. Make sure that their focus is sensitive to the needs of those with eating disorders. Look for groups that are led by a registered dietitian or therapist.

Check out a group by attending two or three meetings before you commit, and be wary of discussions, advice, people, and anything else that triggers your eating-disorder thoughts and behaviors. Attend groups that seem helpful to your recovery, and stay away from those that don't.

Mental Health Therapy

Both the NEDA and International Association of Eating Disorder Professionals foundation (IAEDP) websites have directories to help you find a therapist in your area with specialized training in eating-disorder treatment. If a provider is not available, contact the nearest eating-disorder treatment program that might be able to give you referral information. If the above options leave you empty-handed, either ask your regular medical provider or other professionals for help, or look in your local phonebook under "counseling" to see if anyone advertises experience in treating eating disorders. In beginning therapy, it is important to have some level of comfort with a therapist's knowledge of eating-disorder treatment and a sense of rapport or connection with him or her. Ask about the therapist's eating-disorder education and training, the frequency and amount of continuing education completed on the subject of eating disorders, and how many other clients he or she sees or has seen with eating-disorder issues. Ideally, a therapist will work as a team with your medical provider and nutritionist, so that each professional can focus on his or her role in helping you recover. You can also get the most out of your therapy sessions if you and your therapist focus on the mental health aspects of your recovery and leave the food part to your dietitian.

Nutritional Therapy

You need nutritional therapy with a registered dietitian (RD) who is skilled in treating eating disorders. Ask at your local hospital or eating-disorder program or look in your local phonebook for referrals. If a dietitian also does weight-loss counseling, you may want to ask about what approach he or she would take with your nutritional therapy. Remember, weight-loss counseling, no matter how badly you might want it, is incompatible with eating disorder recovery.

Ask how much training and education the dietitian has in eating-disorder treatment, how many eating-disorder clients he or she has, and what approach he or she uses. Ideally, you should find a dietitian who works with intuitive or mindful eating. There are many sites on the Internet that can help you find a dietitian. Though face-to-face sessions are ideal, it is more important that you find a dietitian skilled in treating eating disorders, and one that you are convinced has a philosophical approach that is in the best interest of your recovery. If there are none in your area, you can find dietitians who do nutritional counseling by phone.

Informal Support

Look around at the people in your life. You can probably identify those who are able to support and help you in the ways that you need support and help. These individuals might be among your immediate family, extended family, and friends. They may be people you know from school, your place of faith, or many other places. Do not let your eating disorder make this decision by choosing help from those who will glamorize or fuel your eating disorder.

Look for those who listen, encourage, talk about emotions more than food, and are not critical about their bodies or yours. It is best if they seem to eat from a mindset that does not include rules about types or amounts of foods that are okay to eat. Talk to them about how they can support you, and decide with them how that support can be put into action. Most of all, be honest with them and teach them what you need and how to give it to you.

People also find sources of strength in members of the clergy, prayer, meditation, knowledgeable lay people, and reading. Make sure that the focus is on healing and forgiveness and not condemnation.

Family Portrait

You know that eating disorders are mind-boggling to most people. Let me remind you that among the many predisposing factors that make a person vulnerable to developing an eating disorder are a highly emotional or sensitive nature, perfectionism, and a personality that strives to do whatever possible to please others. Anyone who focuses on body size, shape and weight, dieting, and critiquing food choices may not be your most powerful ally right now. Validation is important!

You are seeking environmental and family support that can be helpful parts of your recovery. There may be family relationship factors that play a part in your difficulties. If so, in a structured therapy setting, discuss with family members things that they have done, not done, said, or not said that have been hurtful to you. Also, if you have relationships with particular family members where you feel a level of safety that will allow you to hear the same from them, using therapy to address these issues can be valuable as well. The "gold" in this work is in creating an environment where you can seek and make amends, invite and express forgiveness, repair relationships, and make changes where it is possible to do so.

Make decisions about when and how to do these things with care, thought, and the assistance of your therapist, as interactions like this do not always go as planned or desired, and you must be prepared to handle that. You and your therapist can identify those family members who can play an active role in your healing and recovery, and figure out how to teach them how they can help you. Ask them for exactly what you need.

You can also identify family members who may not be the best members for your support team at this time. For example, individuals who struggle themselves, trigger your eating-disorder thoughts and behaviors, or who have difficulty making sense of your eating disorder and are unable to be a consistent source of support for your recovery. In these cases, you may need to work with your therapist to figure out how to navigate these relationships in ways that protect your recovery efforts as much as possible.

Lastly, if there is someone in your family who expresses consistent guilt that he or she may have caused your eating disorder, use caution. You are at risk of hiding your feelings in an attempt to protect this person's emotions. The best thing to do here is to help that family member find a therapist who works with eating disorders and/or a support group. Once you trust that your family member is working to understand and heal his or her pain, you can focus on your own recovery instead of protecting your family member.

 Find someone in your environment with whom you can be honest about your eating-disorder behaviors. Decide how often you will check in with this person, what you will discuss, and how you need him or her to respond. Example: Most of my clients plan a ten-minute check-in with their support person every one to two days. Then write down three to five questions that you will address each time you meet. Examples: Did you binge today? What emotions have you experienced today? What three things did you try to use before you binged? What non-eating disordered behaviors did you use today that were helpful? Did you eat three meals today? Did you do anything to spend calories since we last spoke?

Move forward where you can, as no benefit comes from blaming or guilt. Heal what is realistic and appropriate to heal, with individuals who can help you. You might increase interaction with some family members and decrease interaction with others, based on what is in the best interest of your recovery right now. Make these decisions deliberately, with your therapist, as no benefit comes from rehashing the past or continuously asking, "Why?"

As you gather your troops and train them to help you fight your eating disorder and defend your progress, remember this: you need to find as many supporters as possible. You, like anyone else, cannot be perfect. It is impossible to move toward recovery without mistakes and slips. You must find those with whom you can be honest about what is going on with your eating disorder and your recovery. Your eating disorder will discourage you from being honest when you make mistakes. It is yet another lie that mistakes are something to be ashamed of and hidden. Mistakes are part of recovery, as well as part of being human. Recovery is made up of admitting our mistakes to those who can help us, exploring where we could have done things differently, and making a plan to address it. Recovery is about realizing that you are off track and turning back toward your recovery path, using your growing arsenal of skills, as soon as possible. In fact, that's the best any of us can do when we make mistakes. So gather your troops, train them, have plans to correct tactical errors, and head into battle with your troops around you.

Some days our pain and fear can feel unbearable,
and although our eating-disorder behavior is
also intolerable, it is oh-so-familiar. But there is
another way. We can turn to trusting friends, a
higher power, or a support network in order
to move forward within our recovery.

Today, what we can't do alone we can do together.

8.

Let's Build a New Plan

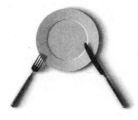

Cold Steel Chairs and the Powerful Truth

By Robyn

Fear is palpable, with the ability to disguise itself in many forms. There was raw fear that would shoot through my body with electrical force and break through every cell of my being until it reached my mind, where it paralyzed me. Then there was the manipulative kind of fear, which had me disguising my truth to get whatever I needed from myself or others so that I could be okay in my own skin. And then there was the enemy I once despised the most and hid from at any cost—vulnerability. Even the thought of having to live through the process of being vulnerable petrified me. It was like sitting on a cold steel chair stark naked on an illuminated stage in front of the whole world, where the lights made my skin transparent, revealing the very heart of me. Vulnerability was unacceptable to me, so I hid.

I hid within my eating disorder. I was not weak or stupid; in fact, I was a clever little thing. I put on my superhero cape and rescued myself from emotions that my pubescent mind could not fathom. My eating disorder was my salvation, the medication that numbed me enough to survive. It provided me shelter from the growing pains of life, and sometimes it even brought me joy and hope. I understand this now.

As a child, the level of discomfort I experienced was something I believed I needed to protect myself from. I am grateful to that little girl for doing all that she could to get me through life. I survived. I thank her. If I were to revisit her, I'd see her in her bedroom bingeing, an act of relief, much like I imagine a hardworking mother might relax with a glass of wine or a magazine after putting her children to bed. She would take a breath: This is her time; she has made it through another day of caring for others. Just as I, the little girl, felt as I stuffed myself with anything I could. I was finding solace, but it was ruined by conflict over ideals and deceptions of what beauty brought. I inherited the perception that "what you look like counts." When my family (including me) teased my father by calling him "Fatty Patty," it seemed so funny at the time, but I also understood it to mean that "fat people" are not respected, and society reflected that daily. He appeared an easy target and willing enough to play along. Later he, too, would seek his comfort, but it was in a six-pack of beer.

The language of this culture was self-taught. At my high school, we were all teenagers who had yet to feel confident in embracing and speaking our true identities. I believe we were all either molding ourselves to fit in or hiding. As with all options, I wanted both, but around the popular loudmouths, I wanted to hide. My round belly, rubbing thighs, and "chubby" cheeks would not let me, as I weaved through the maze of idle students in the corridors to avoid the chant of Phillip Smith and his friends: "Robyn Cruze is a Jenny Craig dropout." I was so embarrassed. I was so ashamed. And the level of fear heightened as I told myself I was in danger of exposing my truth. It felt like I was losing articles of clothing as I frantically tried to reach my scheduled classroom before the rags fell away from my body.

◆ ◆ ◆

My mother's eyes were black, sunken circles, as if she had been beaten with a perfectly circular object. Her body was wilting; we could see her color and vivaciousness drying up before us. There at the dining table at 7 Sadie Avenue, just after I closed my eyes to pretend that my brussel sprouts were ice cream in order to eat them, my mother told us what the doctor had strongly suggested: "I have lupus." By the end of the night, I heard: "I may be dying." These were words she regretted saying to us for the rest of her life. In her own state of vulnerability and fighting for her life as her kidneys threatened to fail, she had spoken the words that changed my life and had me waiting for and dreading her death for nineteen years.

Trauma has a tendency to propel souls into hiding. The debilitating fear of losing my mum played out in my mind like a Brothers Grimm fairytale. I would find myself envisioning her death over and over. In my child's mind, I believed unequivocally that when my mum died, I would die also. I would picture myself—face up, arms spread out across her glossy, black coffin—asking the priest to bury me along with her. I imagined rock particles piercing my flesh as the sun shone through the old gum trees like the hands of God calling out for us both. I had a great need to externalize my emotional pain, and this image satisfied that. Soon after, my binge-purge-starve cycle took that horrid vision's place.

Fear is such a primal thing, a human trait that no one is excluded from. It serves us, as it prepares our bodies to run from danger. But when there is no actual danger and fear begins to dictate our actions and thrust us into greater danger—danger we embrace—there is something wrong. My mum often asked me to do what I knew I needed to do to recover from my eating disorder, just as she did what she needed to do by taking her medicine, changing her diet, and meditating in order to stop the progression of her lupus. Recovery did not stop the fear, shame, guilt, and other negative emotions that come with being human, but it created a safe place for me to examine them, and later put them in their rightful places.

It is said that our truth will set us free. It is the acknowledging of my story and honoring it that has set me free. The little girl in me did what she did to keep me alive; but as an adult, I know better, so I have a choice to do better. It is no longer okay for me to simply survive and dodge my fear. I am a capable woman who now wants to experience life in all its beauty and sometimes ugliness. The shelter of my eating disorder also sheltered me from this full life that I now seek. When I got into recovery, I had to put on the superhero cape and bid farewell to my eating disorder. Its power faded with every truth I began to tell myself, as I redirected my fear to be heard instead of hidden within my eating disorder. Although sometimes it has been difficult not to hide, I have continued to choose comfort in support, pausing, and saying "no" to the quick fix that long ago ceased working for me.

As time goes on, I can still see how my fear gets in the way of things. I wish it wouldn't; it has a terrible tendency to make things so much harder and slow my process down. When I speak from my truth, listen from my truth, question the facts, and let go of the fear, I can move toward a life of freedom that I know has my name on it . . . and sometimes, that's the hardest thing I have to do.

How to Honor Your Fear and Seek Your Truth

By Espra

Being Brutally Honest with Yourself

Eating Disorder: "Robyn had a reason to have an eating disorder. Her mother was dying. You don't have problems like that. You're just weak." Or, if you have had some sort of specific trauma that you can put your finger on, "You are making things up, imagining them as worse than they actually were to justify having an eating disorder."

Truth: Regardless of why your eating disorder came into being, we know that when individuals lack the skills or opportunity within their environments to honor the fact that they have emotional pain, there is an increased risk of developing an eating disorder. Either way, with or without clear traumatic events, individuals needs access to validation by others of the impact of their experiences. In this way individuals learn to validate themselves, increasing their ability to heal from difficult emotional experiences.

Robyn hid. She hid from others and from herself. As with Robyn, it is likely that the vulnerability and honesty you need in order to question the role of your eating disorder and why you need it in your life have become the very enemies you'd do anything to hide from. Being brutally honest with yourself about what your eating disorder brings you (harmful and helpful) can be terrifying. Almost everyone says this as they begin recovery. However, why would an eating disorder have become your solution to coping if you had a less destructive, less complicated way that worked?

Regardless of your personal reasons, know that a function of an eating disorder is to help cope with emotional fear and pain. It offers on a silver platter this "brilliant" solution, as its incessant chatter interrupts and distracts you from more frightening thoughts and emotions. Eating-disorder obsessions and behaviors often bring welcome relief, in a miserably comforting sort of way, as they leave little time or energy to think of other worries. They bring avoidance and distraction. Hope arises as the eating disorder promises lottery-sized returns of true happiness if you embrace it. It may communicate outwardly what you cannot say about hurting inside. There may be other benefits as well. For many, it seems to do a wonderful job, in an immediate sense, before it ultimately robs you of everything.

The eating disorder convincingly presents itself as the only voice of total honesty about your defectiveness and flaws, telling you how to compensate for, conceal, or divert attention from them. It brainwashes you, saying that shoving your body into a particular weight, shape, or size is a brilliant, creative, and unique solution for your dilemmas.

Unique my ass! It is a big fat lie! How about saying, "Brilliant there, eating disorder, a unique solution just for me and eleven million other people in America. You're making me feel pretty special now."

Do you think you don't have a good enough reason to feel emotional pain and fear? This is partly why brutal honesty is so difficult. You may be terrified to admit that you carry emotional pain and burdens, judging yourself and fearing judgment from others that you are weak, wanting attention, or a host of other conclusions. Brutal honesty starts here. It starts with admitting that you carry a burden of emotional pain that scares the crap out of you. No matter how insignificant you think it is, whether you brought it on yourself or it was heaped upon you, whether you deserve it or not, you must take the terrifying step of getting honest about whatever your bottom-line fear might be.

Eating disorders are usually about coping with pain and fear in the best way that you can find. It's safe to assume that if you had the skills to cope with pain and fear outright, you would have done it that way. Most people are not taught those skills, as families rarely know them to teach. You need to stop lying to yourself about why you use your eating disorder. Find your truth and target the bottom line of your illness with a new plan.

What is it that you would like to feel more than anything in the world? Caution: "Skinny, size ___, small enough thighs, cheeks that aren't 'chubby,' not hungry, in control," are not the right answers. Skinny is not an emotion. Fat is not an emotion. As loud, strong, and miserable as they are, they are not emotions; they are thoughts.

Ask yourself, "What is it that I crave to feel more than anything in the world?" When an answer pops into your mind, follow-up with the question, "And if I felt that, what would happen?" Keep asking that question until you get to the bottom of what you really, truly crave. When you believe that you have gotten down to your core emotional craving, write it down. In going through this process, you are showing courage in being vulnerable and honest.

Example: "More than anything in the world I want to feel successful. And if I were successful, what would happen? I'd lose weight. And if I lost weight, what would happen? I'd be skinny. And if I were skinny? I could be outgoing. And if I were outgoing? I could meet people and feel like I belong . . . I would feel included . . . I wouldn't feel all alone." That's it. You wouldn't feel all alone. That's your truth.

You'll know when you get there. You may find yourself sighing, dropping your shoulders, relaxing, or getting teary, to name a few physical clues. The profound words and voice of wise psychodrama expert and teacher, Mary Bellofatto, ring in my head as she once told me, "You know . . . that you know . . . that you know." (Think about that.) Then she said, "And you pretend that you don't know." I've learned through practicing this, both myself and with my clients, that Mary's right. We know when we've hit our core truth, despite often trembling at the thought, and we need to trust it.

The good news is that there are specific skills you can learn to cope with hard emotions without the negative consequences that an eating disorder brings. Please trust that there are more options to living your life than your eating disorder (one extreme) and not acting on your eating disorder in exchange for a life of misery (the other extreme). As you consider this, you, like Robyn, begin to take back your power and use it to build a life worth being a part of.

Question Your Control

Eating Disorder: "With me, you have control over something. You alone control how much or how little you eat or how many calories you do or do not keep in your body. Or you control when you lose control, and that's the ultimate control."

Truth: As we described in Chapter Five, despite the illusion of control, you actually have little to no power in your daily life with an eating disorder. Start owning that truth. You can turn your mindset from control to authentic power by being honest about rituals, binges, purges, nutritional restriction, and other self-destructive activities. Who and what are really controlling your behavior? If the eating disorder is your answer to being in perfect control, why is the power so short-lived?

Eating-disorder behaviors can keep you safe from fear for about as long as it takes to engage in them. Then fear returns. Find safety in learning how to tolerate and regulate your emotions in ways that last beyond the moment. That is the balance that allows a healthy and functional flow of emotions, versus endlessly battling them. They need not become a wall of pressure (that you need more and more eating-disorder behaviors to hold back) or a consuming flood (in which you need more and more eating-disorder behaviors to keep from drowning). As you begin to navigate the water and flow with its current, neither fighting to go faster nor resisting in an attempt to stop, you begin to build skills to cope with emotions and even value them and their intended function of helping you.

The truth is, the more you avoid emotions by using eating-disorder behavior, the more you become convinced that you are incapable of coping in any other way. You do not respond in ways that will keep your emotions and life steady. It is in this way that an eating disorder that seemed to bring perfect control begins to take on a life of its own, making you more and more out of control.

Take a Step Back and Take Back the Power
Eating Disorder: "Honest, I really do help. I numb the pain. Numbing pain is the secret to life . . . and you need me."
Truth: Yes, your eating disorder serves as a quick fix for hard emotions—before it takes everything from you. And it *will* take everything from you.

Take a long, hard look at what you really have control over: yourself, your interests, your journey, your day-to-day behavior, your values, how you interact with and love those around you, and how you show up for life. You are not in control. In fact, you are powerless. Your eating disorder is running your life. If you don't believe me, think about a time when you decided to stop your eating-disorder behaviors. Think about the thoughts and emotions that slammed you as you tried to do it. How long did it last? How long were you able to use sheer willpower and white-knuckle your way through stopping your eating disorder? If not for the eating disorder, would you choose to feel out of control when you eat, exercise so hard or long as to get in the way of other things in your life, spend so much money on food, or put your head into a toilet? When I put it like that, does it spark some doubt about who or what is in control of your life?

The other side of this coin is related to the nature of addiction. People in the throes of addiction, eating disorders included, are convinced their behaviors are veiled in secrecy and affect no one else. This is another lie. Others in your life who are being affected by your mindset and actions are, more than likely, afraid to bring up their concerns about your struggles or the impact of your behaviors on them. Meanwhile, the shame of engaging in such behaviors makes it seem impossible to talk about with others. Thus the veil of secrecy lives on. It is rare that family members, friends, or loved ones of someone with an eating disorder are not aware of some aspect of the illness, are not affected by it, and/ or are not concerned about its effects. Sadly, it is also rare that loved ones can break through their own fears to bring up their concerns about eating-disorder behaviors for discussion. If they do muster the courage to do so, it is rare that eating-disorder sufferers can admit to themselves or others that there is indeed a problem. We just don't know how to talk about the hard stuff. Others do not know how to tell you they are worried that you stay home every night instead of being social, only eat lettuce without dressing, excuse yourself immediately and disappear after eating, or deplete their money or snack food supplies.

Start by getting honest with yourself about the many ways that the eating disorder dictates your life. This will help you get honest about how the eating disorder creates more of the very pain it promises to get rid of.

Get a pen and plenty of paper for writing and make a list. List everything you can recall that you have lied about related to your size, shape, weight, what you have eaten, or what you have not eaten. Write down things you tell others to divert suspicion, plus any instances of betrayal or stealing or violating your own values. Be sure to write down anything that comes to mind that your eating disorder says is not a big deal, for it most likely is.

Examples: "I told my husband that I had to go visit a sick friend so I could binge." "I told my friends that I had a huge exam the next day to avoid eating out." "I told my date that I had already eaten in order to eat as little as possible without it being suspicious." "I stole food." "I stole money to buy food." "I ate food from a dumpster."

Robyn found freedom in being truthful with herself, then with others. As you begin to be honest with yourself about what is actually happening, and then with others you have carefully selected, you begin to heal. The lies and feelings of needing the eating disorder to cope start to fade just a little. As you build a pattern of truthfulness with yourself and then with others, even about your fears, a light will appear in the darkness of the recesses of your heart. Like Robyn, you will feel exposed and want to run to your eating disorder to protect you with its lies. As you redirect your fear and let yourself be heard in safe places, the fear gradually lessens, and you can find comfort in authentic support, learning to see quick fixes and old solutions as fleeting and short-lived. The grand illusion of the eating disorder is that it protects you from pain. The reality is that nothing erases pain for good. Recovery alone does not stop the river of scary emotions any more than changing old, ineffective patterns stops them. Your goal must be to protect yourself by learning to tolerate the pain of these emotions, a process that actually decreases the pain.

Let Robyn's story inspire you to see that allowing yourself to experience the hard emotions that are part of all of our journeys on this earth is what builds the safe container in which to sort, make sense of, and learn to work with them.

Just so you know, fear gets in the way of all of us, me included. I feel validated by Robyn's understanding of what pain does to her, as well as to the rest of us. I feel inspired by Robyn's understanding of how to move beyond it (not to be confused with the myth of making it go away) by accepting that it is there. It is then that we can honor it without getting mired in it, listen to it, understand it, check the facts, and work with it. It is hard to do. But that is true power.

A Word about Shame

Eating Disorder: "You are stupid, fat, worthless, and ugly. You don't deserve to be loved by anyone, and no one would love someone as disgusting as you anyway."

Truth: So many of my clients have said some version of the above statement that it immediately pops into my brain when I think of lies eating disorders tell. How could this be true if you have loved ones in your life? My clients cannot imagine that others with eating disorders might think similarly about themselves. It is an eating-disorder trick— exception to the rule.

In almost two decades of treating individuals suffering with eating disorders, I cannot remember meeting one who does not suffer from shame. Shame plays a big role in the development of an eating disorder. Then shame plays a huge role in perpetuating an eating disorder. It gets to the point where my clients think that everything bad that happens is because they are bad. I challenge the lie by saying something out loud when anything bad happens, like a light bulb going out in my office: "Oh no. That light bulb just went out because you're stupid, fat, worthless, and ugly." Sounds weird put that way, doesn't it? Think about it, though. You do the same thing in your own mind. I just go public with it.

You may feel "eating-disorder" pride in discipline, willpower, self-control; being "better than," competent, talented, clever; or having an identity. You may then feel shame for feeling pride. You may feel shame when you notice happiness, thinking you don't deserve it. You may feel shame for the conflict, lying, pulling away from or pushing away loved ones, loss of control, "weakness," kneeling in front of toilets, or desperation. You may judge yourself or others as "fat and gross," then feel ashamed of yourself for being "superficial." When you chronically feel shame, you isolate, disconnect, and feel unworthy. You might seek comfort in things like bingeing, and then feel shame in violating what the eating disorder insists will make you "thin and beautiful." You may find numbness in not eating or pride in spending calories. But you are lying to those around you in order to do it. Shame increases. I get dizzy thinking about all that spinning.

When shame is allowed to have a mind of its own, it can lead you to withdraw from those who can help you, or with whom you can feel the connection needed for a meaningful relationship and a hopeful and purposeful life. Shame is harming you if you feel a sense of unworthiness about your core nature, are disgusted with yourself, or reject yourself. Then you might do things like insist on perfection from yourself or others, pretend you are perfect, or push away and judge others in the attempt to protect yourself from being judged by them first. These things make eating disorders worse.

Shame probably made it harder to write your response to the last tool. Shame may have gotten you to skip the tool altogether. If the shame is getting in the way of something helpful, see the signals of shame, observe the incoming information, name all that you observe, allow all of it into your mind, then respond deliberately. To help you learn to manage unnecessary shame, as well as eating-disorder thoughts and urges, use this skill to fight back. For example, to decrease shame, go back and wholeheartedly respond to the tool anyway. Shame will make it terrifying to share your responses with a safe, caring person in your life. To decrease shame, identify that person and share with him or her anyway. It is the only way out of the tar pit of shame. This is how you start uncovering your authentic power.

Learn about emotions, understand them, cope and work with them skillfully and effectively. That you can stop or exterminate them with eating-disorder behavior, a body that looks a certain way, or any other attempts to push them down, overpower them, or annihilate them is an illusion—it is not power. Authentic power lies in learning how to face emotions honestly and work with them as they are, in their totality. How could you do this and not feel empowered? Get help and learn how. Instead of spending all of your strength "controlling" emotions because of fear that you will drown in them, you will eventually find authentic power in accepting them, riding with them, and doing what is necessary to navigate those you like and those you don't as just another part of life's journey.

An open heart has me singing silently.
A closed one has me screaming out loud.

A secret buried in fear is fatal to the recovery process.
Open up your heart to others you trust today.
Share your secret anyway, and watch your recovery grow.

9.

Who the Hell Am I, Anyway?

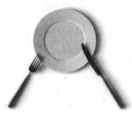

Pizza Nights and Yves Saint Laurent Handbags

By Robyn

Who I was, my identity, had never been enough for me. This was a problem. Because not only was I seeking approval from others (a tool I used constantly to lift my self-esteem), I was also investing in people who could not fix me and placing inappropriate pressure on those I sought to validate me. It was I who had to provide the self-esteem by building it myself. I had to like me. I had to approve of me.

The constant nagging within me of being unworthy and the unshakable feeling that I needed to hustle to have others notice and approve of me was what drove me throughout my life. Beginning to question who I was, what my desires were, and what I wanted to bring to this world was the starting point to finding real joy.

When I was thirteen, I started attending a weekend class for singing, jazz, tap, and drama. It lasted four hours per Saturday. I remember walking up the long set of worn, wooden stairs to the studio where the class was held. I paused on the landing to ask myself, "Who am I going to be today?" Because being me wasn't enough, in order to be okay in my own skin and not spend four hours comparing myself to the other child-star wannabes, I needed to strap on my armor before I hit the foyer. That's where they would be sitting, unavoidable, putting on their tap shoes, singing their practiced lyrics, or stretching for jazz class, where Ms. Georgia took pride in the rapport among her students.

It was not that these highly talented kids planned on hating on me or making fun of me, or even talking behind my back. I'm sure at some point they did these things; I mean, what kid doesn't? Nevertheless, I have no idea how they felt about me for the most part. But try telling a kid with an eating disorder that. It was the stories I told myself that were the true torture. I still have to be mindful of this today.

The true value of recovery is in the process of "checking in" with myself and honoring that voice that longs to be heard and that encourages me to keep moving forward. And with each positive action I take toward this, I secure a little more self-worth from deep within.

After I got over the initial shock in recovery that I really had no idea who I was (I truly had absolutely no idea) and what I liked or disliked outside of my eating disorder, I started to turn it into a game. Sometimes I would try new things and watch how I felt when I was doing them to see if I actually liked them or not.

I found out that I enjoy the rush of flying through the sky hooked to a cable. I love really hot showers, singing out loud, making people laugh, kissing, hiking in the sun with a friend, sleeping, and being heard. These are all vital to my spirit and purpose. I learned I am a social being, but love to curl up by myself with a book after 9:30 p.m. I learned that I like deep conversation, and that idle chitchat like, "So what do you do for a living?" bores me. I learned that

I am a human being who has made bad choices, but I am not a bad person because of them.

I am not my father, nor my bank account, nor my car model; and my worth will never be threatened because of it. I am a human being who has made bad choices, but I am not a bad person because of them. I have learned that I am responsible for my behavior and my thoughts, and that calling for time out when I do not feel comfortable is true self-care. I now believe that clarity comes in a pause, and with that clarity comes a sense of showing up for myself to honor what is trying to call out to me.

I have also learned that just because I know the right way to be or behave doesn't mean I will always choose to do the right action. Sometimes I get angry when I am in fear, exhausted, or hungry. I say things I wish I hadn't, don't exercise when my body is begging me to, and say yes when I want to say no. This is life, and I am learning. I am far from perfect, far from fairytale fantastic, but I am learning to accept my faults with a little more compassion because, and I always come back to this, *I am human.* You see, having acceptance for where I am in the moment doesn't mean that I am excusing inappropriate behavior or not taking responsibility. It means I don't have to go into a panic attack about how horrible I am, and instead I get to move forward . . . most of the time.

I now understand that even when I feel like I can't get through an emotional loss, by going through it, important things will be revealed, and that the way to get through it is to simply show up. I have learned that being a good mother is important to me, but it is not defined by what school my children attend and what clothing brands I buy them. It is defined by the way I show up for them emotionally and how I provide safe boundaries for them to explore. Most of the time hearing them out and letting them know that I see them is often all they need. And usually all I need to get out of my head is to have a cuddle with my daughters. Connection matters to me.

I have learned that my ego (that part of me that needs to be right and the best at all times) is not always my amigo, but that having pride in what I do (that sense of accomplishment in knowing I've done my best) is a wonderful gift to give myself. I have learned that fitting in with others is passé and overrated, that my true friends accept me for who I am, warts and all. It would take a lot for me to lose my best friends, those to whom I long ago bared my soul. For me, friendships are what make this world go 'round. The true connections I experience on my (too infrequent) pizza nights with Andi, Nicole, and Emily are like fuel to my soul. I have learned that Yves Saint Laurent handbags do not define my true character or worth, but they sure are pretty to look at—and if I want to spend my money on them, that's fine with me. I have learned that changing careers does not make the old one a failure or a waste. Change is inevitable in this life, and befriending it removes the need for regrets or "what ifs."

I have learned that when I get quiet and stop trying to force the issue, I can make decisions that best honor me, and in turn, honor all those around me. When I stopped in my tracks and said, "This is who I am; this is my story," I could begin to change and become the woman I had longed to become.

My story was also being revealed within my food. I gained trust in myself, and in turn, my body as I began to allow myself food within a structure that created both freedom and safety for me. Within a short year of brutal honesty with myself, and eating within the safety net of the Structured Approach, I noticed a decreased attachment to my wanting to be perfect that was also mirrored in my food choices. My choices were dictated by my body's need, not the needs of my eating disorder. I learned that the moment I tried to interject my thoughts about food into my body's signals it was bound to throw it into a tizzy, so I don't do that anymore . . . most of the time.

I had long since noticed that I hadn't fluctuated dramatically in weight, or in my emotional state, like I had when I was in my eating disorder. You see, without a binge, there was no substantial weight gain, and all the extra pounds that belonged to the binges had disappeared. I was now at a weight that no amount of dieting in the past had ever sustained. Food no longer plagued me as it once did, simply because it no longer held power. I also noticed that I no longer had the desire to binge or starve because I'd gained wisdom, experience, and truth through my structured eating. I was no longer afraid of my food choices. I knew through my experience with the

Structured Approach that weight gain was due to eating when I was not hungry or past being full and not as intricately gauged by the choices I made. I found that the choices I made were now in direct proportion to how much fuel I needed and whether I actually liked the food I was eating. I was also at ease with dining out. I was more comfortable listening to what my body wanted to eat, and noticed that it was from that voice that I usually made my food decisions. My body had organically moved into a Mindful Approach; and this time, it was my mind that followed. I had turned a corner in my recovery.

The Mindful Approach was a process that I had been naturally practicing within the Structured Approach for many months. I wrestled a little with letting go of the structure, but I reminded myself that I could always go back to it if I felt, at any stage, unsafe. There is a magical freedom around food within the Mindful Approach. The obsession has long since been lifted, and the trust in myself and my choices took the eating disorder's place. Yes, sometimes I still have a weight conscious thought. But when this occurs, it is more like a little buzzing in my ear that I can shoo away than a sledgehammer to my brain. My food choices became about aligning to my truth and strength, and the woman I want to become. My plate now tells a very different story from what it did with the eating disorder. The eating disorder doesn't visit anymore.

Pizza, Handbags, and Beyond

By Espra

Get Quiet
Eating Disorder: Blah, blah, blah . . .
Truth: The eating disorder says nothing new. It just shows up. It is predictable, belligerent, and won't shut up long enough to let you hear yourself think.

Deep honesty with yourself and trusted others continues to be a crucial part of your recovery. The eating disorder's relentless harassment and mandates are possibly all you have been able to hear and think about for quite some time. Trying "not to think about it" works about as well as that old game where you "try not to think about pink elephants" for one minute. It can't be done. Obeying your illness's mandates rewards you with a brief moment of peace from its constant reminders about your defectiveness and flaws. It has become your life. Your eating disorder might now even be your identity.

Recovery involves finding ways, other than obeying your illness, to slow down that eating-disorder voice. It starts with creating one fleeting moment of silencing the voice, or at least decreasing its volume. With time and practice, you can tone down or silence the voice for longer periods. The unique current of your recovery will determine how quickly this shift happens. Your job is to practice as much as possible so as not to hold back the flow. Research shows that a consistent practice of choosing where you place your attention, noticing when it has wandered, and bringing it back to the intended object of your focus helps you cultivate the skill to refocus and quiet unwanted thoughts and urges. Resources for learning about and practicing these mindfulness skills can be found in a number of places, including Eastern mindfulness traditions like meditation and yoga, and activities created specifically to train your brain in targeted ways.

As you cultivate your ability to focus your mind, it begins to get quiet. Like Robyn found, the pauses make way for clearer thinking that helps you hear the voice of your own wisdom and intuitive knowing, then separates it from the eating-disorder voice. That is how we all wake up, listen, and start to honor our authentic selves. It happens as you take one glimpse at a time into the frightening and peaceful stillness in between and beyond your habitual thoughts. The longer the pauses, the more you can see—in the words of a friend of mine, "That which brings a different possibility of the knowing of the self."

Check In with Yourself
Eating Disorder: "Ha. Funny. What self? There's nothing there to check in with. That's why you have me."
Truth: When your thoughts, emotions, goals, and identity are wrapped around an eating disorder, there's no way to figure out what could be there.

The eating disorder tells you it is the only place for you to get honest feedback about your shortcomings. It convinces you that by controlling food or the size of your body, you will measure up. Pay attention. You need to be brutally honest with yourself about your goodness. My clients say, "Argh! Espra, you just don't quit, do you?" I reply, "No. This is life or death, and I will always fight for your life." To catch the eating disorder lying about your goodness, watch for those all or nothing thoughts. Maybe you are beginning to recognize them as red flags that the eating disorder is directing your thoughts. Catch it in the act of convincing you that you are all bad or unworthy. Really? Is it actually possible for anyone to be either all (as in 100 percent) bad or all good? Yeah, yeah, you are an exception to the rule. I hope you have a fleeting thought that questions this lie as well.

For survival purposes, all of our brains are made for difficult and intense things to stick and tumble around while pleasant things more frequently slip out. In survival situations this is useful but otherwise it can be miserable. It is frustrating that the authentic voice of encouragement, wisdom, and intuition whispers quietly and the eating-disorder voice shouts its demands at full volume. It takes awareness and practice to tune in to the authentic voice. Each time you attend to the voice of your authentic self, it is like watering a plant. It will eventually take root, and you will start to see and appreciate it as it makes its way through the soil and manure and heads for the light. Then you can begin to align your behavior with that voice, moving closer to the peace we find when we look within for fulfillment, instead of looking outside ourselves.

Look carefully for thoughts or ideas that feel true and real to you, and watch out for those you think you are "supposed" to have, those you "shouldn't have," those that scare you, those that you think you cannot achieve, those you think you don't deserve. You will need to carefully consider your values, your likes, your dislikes—everything that you believe in. Robyn found a helpful way to do that by checking in with her body.

Try this: Think of one thing that you know you like, perhaps a color. Then think of a color you know you don't like. Now look at each color for a while and notice the sensations in your body. Sensations give you cues about your true likes and dislikes.

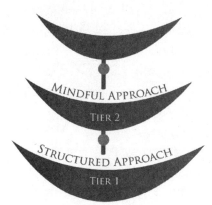

NUTRITIONAL HEALING: A 3-TIER APPROACH™

Start to Consider Tier Two of the Three-Tier Approach to Nutritional Healing: The Mindful Approach to Eating

Eating Disorder: "Skip this section. You already know when you are hungry and full."

Truth: Your eating-disorder thoughts tell you when you are hungry and full. Think about its agenda. You can't trust the eating disorder's information if you are going to recover from it. However, your body is not an accurate informant for nutrition right now either. It is off balance, out of practice, and generally confused about hunger and its nutritional needs.

If you want to consider alternatives to being the prisoner of an eating disorder, you will need to get honest about the most terrifying thing that you could possibly face—food and eating. Getting honest about when you are physically hungry and when you are physically full begins to loosen the control of the eating disorder over you. The challenge is to be honest about when, what, and how much food your *body* is telling you it physically needs and wants. Robyn calls

Getting honest about when you are physically hungry and when you are physically full begins to loosen the control of the eating disorder over you.

this "listening to your body's mind." It is the antithesis of listening to the eating disorder's mandates. You must become aware of and override prior learning—rules about food types and amounts, thoughts about when and why to start eating and stop eating. Even if you are reading this book and do not have an eating disorder, some of the thoughts and emotions that lead you to eat or not eat might surprise you: "It's been a hard day. I am tired and stressed. I deserve to relax with my favorite ice cream." Or "It's been a hard day. Forget eating. I deserve a vacation from having to think about food or eating for the rest of the day."

It took Robyn about a year of using the Structured Approach to eating before she was able to maintain her own safety around food and trust her body enough to allow it to guide her eating, despite her thoughts, rules, or fears. Consider the time you spend with the Structured Approach like learning to walk a tightrope. It provides an anchor to train your balance, with a safety net beneath you. You gain trust in yourself, your choices, and your body based on the skills you are using, rather than the deceptions of your eating disorder. It takes time to stabilize your body physically, to increase your capacity for thinking logically about alternatives, as well as to stabilize preoccupation with food. It takes time to stabilize your fears about eating, what food will do to you, "losing control," and feeling satiated. It takes time to restore your metabolism, your body's optimal functioning, and a more balanced lifestyle in general. It takes time to restore your body's ability to register nutritional information and give signals to your brain based on that. If you try to move beyond the Structured Approach before all of these things are more stable, you may run into hopelessness and despair. You can find yourself restricting nutrition or bingeing because your body is not yet stable and skilled enough to use its own wisdom in a way that supports recovery.

Recovery cannot be rushed, as the price of falling without a safety net is high. Robyn and I feel that a minimum of one year with the Structured Approach makes sense. Determine with your dietitian how long you need to use a structured eating plan before you have the skills to meet the challenge of a more flexible plan.

Only then will the Mindful Approach to eating benefit you. The Mindful Approach has structure, but less than the Structured Approach. You will begin to choose what, when, and how much to eat, surrounded by the safety net of eating regular meals and snacks to meet your body's physical and chemical needs. If you are not hungry at all, regardless of the reason, it is still important to keep some structured intake, but you may choose to eat less than when you are hungry.

In the past few years more resources have become available to help you learn ways to practice eating mindfully. An amazing resource to help you better understand what mindful eating entails as well as tools for approaching it is the groundbreaking book, *Intuitive Eating* by Evelyn Tribole and Elyse Resch. Education and your own dietitian are the best resources to help you supplement your information for this phase of your recovery.

The Mindful Approach is about paying careful attention to your cravings, the flavors of food, how your experience changes as you eat, and when food becomes less enjoyable to your taste buds, instead of paying attention to your thoughts and emotions. One way to practice this type of mindfulness is to observe where on your tongue you taste different flavors. Taste buds that pick up different flavors, such as salty, sweet, or spicy, are clustered in different places on your tongue. You move away from ideas of "good" and "bad" foods and let your body choose a wide variety of foods that sound good, rather than a narrow range of "safe" foods and amounts. Consider additional personal variables as well. For example, some medications can block the brain's ability to register when you have had enough to eat. To mindfully eat, you may have to monitor the physical sensations of pressure and fullness in your stomach to indicate when you are full because your brain won't tell you when you've had enough to eat.

 To prepare for the Mindful Approach, identify your (versus your eating disorder's) food likes, dislikes, and cravings. You must understand the thoughts, habits, emotions, and beliefs that all have a part in your relationship with food. Start by making a detailed list of every thought, rule, feeling, belief, and habit that directs your choices about when to eat, what or what not to eat, and how much. Be specific. Then go back through your list several times to add things you initially missed.

Example: 1) I am stressed out. I want to relax with my favorite ice cream. I choose the flavor and amount based on my desire to relax with ice cream instead of sensations in my belly or on my taste buds. 2) I feel stressed and anxious. I don't want the hassle of choosing, preparing, or eating food, so I don't eat. 3) If I eat more than others, I am a pig, so I make sure I eat less than them. Then I go home and binge. 4) If my stomach is growling and it's mid-morning, I can't eat because it's not yet noon. So I have more coffee. 5) I love fresh bread. I have to eat all I can before it is gone. I start my diet again on Monday. 6) It is wasteful not to eat everything on my plate.

• •

No one perfects mindful eating because no one, not even monks, can be mindful 100 percent of the time. I'll bet that even monks overeat sometimes. Sometimes you will become overly hungry or overly full. Eating unmindfully in one instance does not equate to failing at mindful eating; it is human because it is an ongoing "practice." We wake up, notice that we are not mindfully eating, and then return to the Mindful Approach as soon as possible. It is a process. We remember that each moment is a brand-new chance to make a different choice. Sometimes we notice, yet we don't want to do it differently. This is an opportunity to take a look at what emotion, thought, or belief might be driving the behavior and consider our options. The Mindful Approach is made up of a set of skills that we must strive to continually develop and honor with practice and time. It cannot be perfected. It is difficult. It is liberating.

Deserving and Worth
Eating Disorder: "You don't deserve to eat. You don't deserve to enjoy food. You don't deserve to recover. You don't deserve to be happy."
Truth: This is how eating disorders operate for most people. As you've read, Robyn's drove her to go to extraordinary lengths to earn the approval of others.

The lies come at you with a vengeance, like arrows at a target. They pierce your mind and your heart, driving into you that you are nothing without an eating disorder, nothing but an invisible "other" or someone who takes up too much space in a crowd, and deserves nothing more. They convince you that you will never stand out as unique, interesting, or appealing because there is nothing special about you. You don't deserve to eat; you don't deserve to stop eating; you don't deserve to be free of punishment (even if you have to continue it yourself with the help of your humble servant, the eating disorder). Catch these lies!

My clients are certain they are the only ones in the world who feel inadequate, unworthy, or unlovable. They are not. Robyn was not, and you are not. Keep paying skeptical attention to that eating-disorder voice. As you try to pull away, it will bounce back. Keep talking back to it. It doesn't have to be your identity. Right now you are starting to piece together your own identity aside from the eating disorder, and we are helping you get started.

Do you live in fear that unless you are perfect, someone will see through your facade, exposing the truth that you are a fraud, an empty shell? Are you convinced that most people judge you negatively and see you as "less than," even if they won't admit it? Does it seem like you were born defective, but can't put your finger on exactly how? Does anything here sound familiar? Your eating disorder loves this stuff. If I were filled with a cold, dark, consuming certainty that I was defective, I wonder if I might go to any lengths, maybe even self-destructive ones, to get away from it as well.

Most everyone feels varying degrees of this. You read it right. I know, I know . . . the difference is that *they* aren't defective and *you* are. Busted, eating disorder! It is using an exception to the rule. You are special only in a negative way, or so it tells you. It is so common for people to fear being exposed as a fraud that it has a name: "Imposter Syndrome." For instance, I am convinced that people often think I am more competent and know more than I really do. If they knew the truth about what I do and do not know, they would know I'm a fraud. People might tell me otherwise, but they are just being nice. Robyn has confided in me that she has the same feelings. But how can Robyn be silly enough to think that about herself? She is amazing.

Use this information to question your eating disorder. Ask around, check the facts, consider the evidence, and use those to draw a logical conclusion.

Feeling unworthy can lead to extreme efforts to be perfect as a way to earn value and worth. The problem is that imperfection is the human condition. Human beings are bound to break any streak of perfection because that's how we (you included) are made. The eating disorder says you must rise above imperfection in order to be good enough. This comes at a great cost to you, your time, your relationships, and your life. Is the picture of the craziness of eating-disorder expectations getting any clearer?

Human beings are bound to break any streak of perfection because that's how we (you included) are made.

Even when you get a fleeting sense of being worthwhile as a result of being the "best" at restricting your nutrition, spending unwanted calories, eating "healthy," being the perfect size or weight, it is temporary. That is the transient nature of using outside measures to define your worth or value. It is like winning the big prize at a carnival game. You are good, you are the best, and everyone can see it. Then you see someone with the same prize. You are deflated. The feelings of inadequacy rise up, and you feel compelled to go back, spend your money, and be the best again. The real question here is how much satisfaction do you get from having a life-sized stuffed panda in your room at home? And how long will that satisfaction last?

Figuring Out What Makes You Tick

Eating Disorder: "Look, just get everything else done first and then you'll have time to sit around and think about anything you want."

Truth: As you get quiet and honestly consider your essence, you begin to get glimpses of your interests, talents, and strengths. You haven't had the mental space to attend to such matters thanks to the eating disorder's chatter and illusions. First things first: the best way to run back to your eating disorder for security and comfort is to believe that your only choices are the extremes of figuring out who you are all at once or living in isolation behind your painful mask of "safety" with your eating disorder.

Question these illusions; that's what recovery is made of. Figuring out who you are is a long, ongoing process. For Robyn, beginning to question her desires and deciding what she wanted to bring to the world was a part of her early path to finding true peace. Robyn wasn't *finding* self-esteem, she was *creating* it based on her authentic desires, passions, values, and goals, while creating day-to-day actions that lined up with those desires, passions, values, and goals. You likely have either lost these parts of yourself or never known them at all. Expect to feel terrified that there is no "self" to be found. Try to focus instead on how to build yourself up. Self-esteem is built from each positive action that supports a part of your authentic self. Each action that you take toward supporting those parts of your authentic self builds your foundation by securing your self-esteem from deep within.

 Make a list of sixty-seven things that you think you might like to learn or experience before you die. Leave nothing out because it seems too big, too small, or out of reach. If you run out of things to put on your list, which you will, add smaller steps toward some items and add "stupid little things." Choose one item from your list that you want to pursue first. List all of the steps you would have to take to make that particular goal real for you. If you feel overwhelmed after listing the steps, go back and insert smaller steps between the larger ones. Keep breaking down each step until it feels doable. All steps are possible when you break them down enough. Make sure the goal is your own, and make the steps toward your goal enjoyable and interesting to you. Sixty-seven lines are a lot to fill. Stay with it; keep coming back to it and get through it any way you can. It does not and cannot be "perfect," "right," or even entirely accurate. It just has to stimulate your brain to consider the possibilities. I promise, neither Robyn nor I will hold you to any single thing you write on this list. If you are going to create a life outside of your eating disorder, you absolutely need a list!

Example: 1) Goal: Jump on a bed. 2) Goal: Backpack in Volcanoes National Park. Steps: Find Volcanoes National Park on a map. Read about it on the Internet. Go to a bookstore, sit down with a beverage, and look through travel books. Look up airfares. Make a list of ways to set aside money.

●●

If you notice yourself thinking that some of the items on your list are "stupid," too big, too small, unattainable, unacceptable, not feminine or masculine enough, against the wishes of someone else, wishful thinking—write them down anyway. It is the only way to tap into your authentic desires. Some will go against what others want for you, what they think is okay, or what you "should" want or do. There will be others that you believe you want because you are "supposed" to want them. Write those down also. This is the kind of honesty I am talking about. It is hard to write down what you think you like or want when you have no earthly idea what these things might be. Warning: No eating-disorder goals allowed.

Most of us have heard stories about people getting inspired to run out and do all of the things they've always wanted to do before they died. You are in the opposite situation. It is as if you have been dead, at least inside, and you are now hustling to think of everything you always wanted to do when you woke up. This act will wake you up. This will begin to develop in you an authentic sense of self, identity, and worth.

Ruling Out What Doesn't Make You Tick
Eating Disorder: "Go ahead. Make their stupid list. Just write things ... anything. It doesn't matter. You are hollow, shallow, and so dull that there's nothing to find no matter how many things you write on a piece of paper."
Truth: Yes, go ahead and write just anything. Figuring out who you are is done by experimenting with many things to learn both what you like and what you don't like.

For once, let's just go along with that eating-disorder voice. You jumped through the hoop and made your list just to say that you made a list. What happens if you set out to experiment with items on it and have to scratch them off because you find you don't like them or they are things that someone else wanted you to dream? To find answers to the "Who the hell am I, anyway?" question, you will need to experiment with the things on your list, getting a sense for what you like and want to explore further versus what you don't like. It can be as fun to scratch items off your list as it is to discover what you want to continue to pursue. Right here, right now as you are considering this, you are learning who you are, partly through learning who you are *not*. And that's the way it's done. My "Life Goals" list (posted in my planner so I can always keep them in mind) once had skydiving on it. Today I am certain I would not enjoy skydiving. I think I like the riverboat ride at Disneyland better.

It can be helpful to say your eating disorder's answers to the "Who the hell am I?" question out loud. (I'd suggest doing so somewhere private, since you will be talking to yourself.) "Who the hell am I?"

"I am an eating disorder. That's who I am."

"Who am I?" "I am a fat, lazy slob who can't stop eating."

"Who am I?" "I am the one with enough self-discipline to eat salad with no cheese or dressing (and talented enough at acting to convince others that I like it that way)."

"Who am I?" "I am clever enough to devise a million reasons to skip a meal."

"Who am I?" "I am the math wizard who calculates how many calories I've ingested and how much exercise it takes to burn them (plus a little more)."

Say these answers aloud and really listen to them. In the words of a past client, "Congratulations, I am the very best at something (disordered eating) that matters the very least in life."

Check Your Ego at the Door

Eating Disorder: "If you control what you eat well enough, you can finally be good enough for people to accept and approve of you. *Then* you can be proud of yourself."

And,

Eating Disorder: "How dare you feel proud of anything you've done? How conceited. You should be ashamed of yourself for being so haughty and prideful."

Truth: I'm calling "twisted logic, eating disorder," on this one. Remember the illness's love for using two sides of the same coin to argue its point? When you catch it in the process, it can tip you off that it's out to win, no matter what, and that, in the words of a past client, "ED's messing with your head."

My clients struggle with the idea of pride, often believing that it is egotistical and wrong. Some of us are taught this. Depending on where you look to find a definition of pride, it can look like either a desirable or an undesirable character trait. However, when you live in a way that aligns with your long-term goals and values, a sense of self-acceptance and inner peace starts to take root. It is different from the pride you experience when others or the eating disorder give you approval. This pride moves you toward a sense of self-respect, self-esteem, or satisfaction because of what you are doing. Then it moves into pride about who you are, and, although it will feel strange, there is nothing wrong with that kind of pride.

Stop Trying to Fit In

Eating Disorder: "Duh. If you weren't such a misfit, others would accept you, and you wouldn't have to work so hard to fit in. But you are. So you do."

Truth: People do tend to quickly lose interest when you describe your most exciting endeavor as having the "self-discipline" to resist donuts, or lack of willpower to resist them or get rid of the calories after eating them. What your eating disorder ignores is that you have nothing interesting to say about your life, what you are doing, your dreams or goals because your eating disorder is your life and your eating disorder is boring!

Trying to be who you think others want you to be so they will accept you is extremely limiting and costly. You cannot always choose the people you want to have in your life. When you believe you must be what others want so they will accept you, you become enslaved to winning approval and attempting to read people's minds to predict who they want you to be. You might spend your life waiting to be chosen (for friendships, careers, romance) by whoever will have you.

What if you had an alternative? What if you began to identify and create experiences around your goals and interests, rather than around which foods you resisted or consumed, or efforts to control your body? What if you looked around in your world, found, and surrounded yourself with others who have similar likes, interests, goals, and values? You just might feel some acceptance, and acceptance is more enduring than approval. Perhaps this approach might seem to bring things other than misery to your life.

Start tuning in to hear the whispers of your internal voice. Expect there to be fear that only a worthless core or empty shell will be exposed when you try this new type of focus. Then tune in to it anyway. Remember the time and energy you have invested in an effort to hide your core being. It takes your eating disorder to cover it up. And it makes you miserable. A mentor of mine says eating-disorder thinking says, "Who do I need to be for you to approve of me?" Recovery thinking says, "This is who I am. I hope you are okay with that." Thus begins the life-long journey of discovering who you are.

> The ride is much more fun when you let go.
> There are times when we feel like we are hanging
> on to anything that will hold us up and safeguard
> us from the roller-coaster of life and its emotions—
> like our diet, our body size, and the story we tell
> others. But the truth is, life is a journey, and there
> is no safeguarding ourselves from anything.

Today I will let go of fear. I will let go of the expectation that the eating disorder can and will safeguard me from being hurt. I will embrace the unknown and let go, enjoying the ride of life.

10.

Speak Out. Speak Your Truth. Speak Strong!

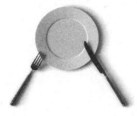

Gushing Rivers and Shocking Phone Calls

By Robyn

Fear of my secrets dissolved the more I spoke them. The more I spoke them, the more they lost their power. The more I witnessed the lack of their power, the more my sense of self grew. This is what ultimately replaced the cycle of my eating disorder.

One of the most challenging things about recovery was learning how I really felt about things. I was so used to trying to please others, or delegating the responsibility to other people to make decisions, that I had lost connection and trust with my own truth. Often I would find myself just nodding my head when someone in a social situation would say something. I feared looking and feeling stupid. Within most conversations where strong opinions were involved and others seemed adamant about what they were saying, I figured they were right, and nodding prevented me from having to partake in the conversation. I got by for many years on my acting skills.

With my loved ones, I often spoke from both sides of my mouth. I would find myself becoming angry if Tim wanted to comment about something I said. I took his need to comment as a challenge to catch me out. The statements he questioned were made up of disjointed resentments, fears, and judgments that had built up each time I had not put a voice to them. They ran out of my mouth like water gushing from a river that had been blocked by a boulder—sometimes raging and damaging. When the boulder is removed, the force and speed causes the river flow to be powerful and choppy, just like the combination of my thoughts and emotions. My practice of saying nothing in order to get through uncomfortable conversations without causing waves was now causing floods.

Often in our household, I said things I thought Tim wanted to hear. I wanted him to love me, approve of me, and want to be with me. Because of this habit, there was no honoring of my truth and I had no self-worth as a result. I couldn't understand why he wanted to question things that I had only said because I thought he wanted to hear them. Was it because I didn't believe what I was saying, so neither did he? I believe now that Tim didn't believe me because I didn't believe me. But in order to change that, I needed to speak from my truth—so that this truth could form a solid foundation for our relationship—not from the unstable dishonesty that had only been propping it up. But speaking my truth frightened me.

I didn't want to be disliked, and I didn't want to be accountable or place boundaries in relationships where there had never been any. But then I had to ask, "What have I done in my life that was so horrible that I cannot trust myself to speak?" And there it was, as clear as day: I have done nothing wrong, except to place the expectation on myself that I should know everything and be everything to everyone. When I brought this expectation to my awareness and asked myself if I would put the same expectation on anyone else, I almost laughed out loud at the absurdity of it all. I started asking myself what I was running from when I did not speak my truth. What kind of relationships was I setting up for myself if they were based on a character that was so far removed from who I really was? The recognition of this truth gave me the power to start speaking it.

When I was in treatment, an extended family member questioned my motives in having my girls come to visit me. He and his wife were minding our girls during the days while Tim was at work, and they were attempting to soothe our toddlers' hearts by telling them that I had gone on vacation to Australia to visit my family. Although I knew their comments to my girls came from a place of love, it was simply unacceptable to me that my children believed I went to Australia without them. The truth was that their mommy was very unwell and suffering from depression and using alcohol to soothe herself, and by going to treatment, she was looking after herself so she could be a better mommy. I called my treatment "Mommy Camp." It was a camp that I truly needed to get through the trauma, break the cycle of depression by learning how to maintain mental health, and learn how to self-soothe without using substances. It is in the asking for and getting help that not only helps us, but also all those around us.

It is in the asking for and getting help that not only helps us, but also all those around us.

When it was time for my girls to visit me, the extended family member, who I believed to care for me and with whom I felt I had a fairly good relationship, contacted the treatment center directly to question the decision my therapist and I had agreed upon to have the girls visit. I believe now that his action was motivated by a desire to protect them emotionally, and in that he chose not to speak to Tim or me before doing so, and instead contacted a friend of a friend who worked there. In treatment facilities, staff members must have patients' written consent to even comment on whether patients are in the facility or not. The staff could not respond to the concerns he raised. What they did do is have my counselor encourage me to deal with the fact that my extended family member was questioning a decision the staff and I had come to (to have my girls visit), a decision that we knew to be in the best interest of my children, my husband, and myself. Oh wow. I had to get on the phone and ask my family member if there was something I could tell him in response to his call. I so appreciated the support of the two staff members sitting close by as he told me I was being selfish and that he had never liked me because we were "oceans apart." Even after that call when attempting to clarify his words, which I thought I must have misinterpreted on the first call, during a phone therapy session with my counselor, he stated that he "didn't care for me," I had to sit with this shocking information. For it was *his* truth, and what our relationship truly was when the smoke and mirrors had collapsed. And as shocking as it was to me (I really had no idea), it was wonderful!

After that phone call and resulting therapy session, I began to sit with the truth that someone didn't like me, and I couldn't do anything about it. A truth that I thought was unbearable. And I survived it. It gave me permission to stop acting in that relationship, and to stop saying things that were not true just so he would like me. I believe I now speak my truth to him, although it took a while for me to feel comfortable around him again. I have boundaries in that relationship when it comes to topics of conversation in which I choose to participate now. Some things I feel comfortable speaking to him about, and some things are uncomfortable, unnecessary, or even harmful for me to share. You see, I don't have to pay the price of sacrificing my honesty and my self-respect by trying to control whether or not he approves of me; I no longer need his approval in order to feel okay about myself. What I do require is that he honors and respects the gift of being a part of my daughter's lives, and he truly does this with great love. Today, I am not the confused woman who was trying to be everything to everyone and losing herself in the process. So while I'm still not certain if he likes me or just tolerates me—either way, I'm in acceptance with the way it is, because I'm in acceptance of me.

No one had ever told me that "I don't know" was an acceptable answer to a question. Or even, "I'm not sure about that, can I get back to you?" I always had a sense that I had to respond in a flash. I had what I now like to call "self-imposed urgency." I believed that taking the time to think about my responses showed people that I had no idea about things. I was so busy trying to protect an image I thought others wanted to see and to which they would be attracted. They wanted to see "the woman behind the curtain," and instead I gave them "the almighty Oz." I ultimately lost many business relationships due to this mentality, and many intimate ones as well.

I thought shooting from the hip was quirky and admirable, but how I chose to use those traits was inappropriate, and was only a reflection of my fear and low self-worth. Looking back, my relationships with my best friends were rarely affected because I always spoke my truth with them, and that was more than enough for them. So it had to be enough for me. My job in recovery became about unlocking my truth, then speaking and acting from it. The fear of "What will happen if I do so?" diminishes with the reality of what actually happens when I have done so.

As I pretended to be a waiter as I served my girls their breakfast this morning, they corrected me in my play when they said I was supposed to take the menus away. Jokingly, I said, "Okay! Stop bossing me!" Lilly's based-on-fact response: "I'm just teaching you how to be a waiter, because you don't know." And although it was a joke, she was right. My unconscious perception that people are out to get me and that I need to know everything is still alive, even though it no longer serves me in my new life.

I continue to learn that to withhold my truth is to withhold intimacy and connection. But truth starts with self. On this journey of recovery, facing my truth, my story, my life as it is— with all its confusion, shades of emotions, faults, passions, and humanness—is enough. I have learned that when I speak my truth, I also give others the permission to speak theirs, just like my extended family did. Today I do my best to take pride in my responses to others. Today, my truth is enough. If you don't like it, it is none of my business. One thing is for certain though, as the saying goes, "the truth will set us free."

How to Stand Still in a Current

By Espra

Unlock Your Truth
Eating Disorder: "You're fat and undisciplined. That is your truth. I'm just telling you the truth because no one else will."
Truth: This is not truth. This is name calling. This is verbal abuse. Hopefully no one in your life calls you names, and if anyone does, hopefully you can get away from him or her.

As you practice listening beyond the eating disorder's lies to uncover your authentic desires, you develop the capacity to see yourself honestly. At this point, you will be well into your own recovery journey. You are unlocking your own truths. You start to look at who you really are, and gradually decrease your dependence on your eating disorder to define, hide, or perfect you. You challenge the urge to let your fear keep you mute. You begin to peel off parts of the eating-disorder mask to slowly reveal what's behind it—your authentic thoughts, feelings, and preferences. And yes, you feel terror because you risk losing something that's been so important you would lay down your life for it—your illness, which promised the approval of others so you could feel accepted, and thus worthwhile.

Courage comes after we do what we are afraid to do.

Living your truth takes courage. You won't trust it yet. Keep doing it, and self-trust will begin to sneak up on you. Remember, courage comes after we do what we are afraid to do. This is how you will begin to trust yourself. It is the opposite of denying your feelings, hiding, and people-pleasing. A difficult truth is that you are not perfect, never will be, and no attempts to control your size, shape, or eating will make you so. And you are worthwhile, acceptable, and lovable anyway.

You know by now that eating disorders are driven by shame, and guilt loves to go along for the ride. Then, in turn, eating-disorder behaviors like lying, deception, and violating your values increase the shame and guilt. The intertwined connection of each to the other takes you further down the slippery slope of misery. A large part of recovery is about decreasing the shame and isolation that both cause and are perpetuated by the hiding and dishonesty. Looking beyond the shame helps you see from all angles of honesty to help you block the eating disorder's hold on you. Otherwise, the illness can block you by convincing you that you are being forthright and honest when it is only partially the case. Dishonesty can take multiple forms. To consider the full spectrum of your behavior, values, and beliefs about honesty, it is helpful to ask yourself whether or not your idea of honesty includes the following: answering a direct question truthfully; what you leave out or don't say; knowing that a person believes something that is not true or complete and allowing them to continue believing it anyway.

It helps to consider shame when you are considering the question of honesty with others. It is not best to set about being indiscriminately and totally honest with everyone. That can backfire, and your eating disorder will be thrilled to remind you that it was right. Getting honest with others begins with creating as much safety as possible. Begin to unlock your truth by preparing to discuss it with someone who is unlikely, based on concrete evidence, to reject you because of it. Of course you won't feel 100 percent safe as you embark on this task, so it is important to create as much structure and safety as possible to allow you every possible advantage.

 Consider the people in your life, such as therapists, parents, siblings, extended family, friends, leaders, clergy, and support groups. 1) Make a list of people to whom it might be safe to reveal parts of yourself. These are people with whom there is a low risk of rejection. 2) For each person, write down the facts: What have you personally seen that person do or heard that person say that will provide evidence about whether or not he or she will hold information about you in a nonjudgmental and safe manner? Use this information to draw factual conclusions about those who might be the least likely to reject you based on what you disclose to them.

For example, your aunt eats mindfully, never talks about dieting, forbidden foods, or disliking her body or others' bodies. Those facts logically suggest that she would be a safe person with whom to discuss your eating disorder. In contrast, you hear a particular friend repeating things others have told her in confidence. She would not be a safe person to confide in. Even if she says she will protect your truths you see her actions and hear her speak otherwise. The risk is high that she will do the same with you. Again, make sure that the people you eliminate from consideration are rejected based on actual evidence, and not from your shame or fear.

Also, make sure you choose individuals who are not likely to reinforce your eating-disorder thinking, who will not expect you to be perfect in order to be good enough, and who will hold you accountable for not staying honest.

• •

Use factual information to make your decisions instead of relying exclusively on thoughts, feelings, or other things you happen to make up. Making decisions based on the latter criteria leaves the door wide open for your eating disorder to flood into your thinking, your feelings, and your actions. By using facts, you deal with the reality of what is helpful in the moment. Facts are the great enemies of the eating disorder, as they will always expose its lies.

Speak from Your Truth
Eating Disorder: "Whatever. Try their honest approach, tell people everything about you, and watch what happens. You'll be sorry."
Truth: Extremes are a tool of the eating disorder. Honesty does not mean telling people everything, as that is just as dangerous as totally hiding your self, thoughts, and feelings.

Like Robyn, you will find that the power of your secrets and shame decreases as you speak of them where it is safe to do so. Gather concrete evidence about how many people jump up and run out of the room screaming because of what you reveal. Use the facts that you gather as ammunition against the eating disorder's lies. A crucial element of using behavior that is contrary to your shame is to do it "all the way." In DBT we teach clients how to guide their facial expressions, posture, and tone of voice, and speak up as if they have nothing to be ashamed of. Because behavior and posture can quickly change the way your brain processes and continues to create emotions, doing the opposite of shame opens the way for shame to decrease. Then different emotions can arise that might be more tolerable as well as useful in the situation.

Speaking your truth helps you take care of yourself and the relationships in your life. When we suppress our thoughts, feelings, needs, and wants, we build resentment and tension on both sides, and things blow up or fall apart. Truth-telling is critical to finding and keeping healthy, supportive relationships in your life. It also helps keep relationship drama and blow-ups from running rampant. In your eating disorder, there are ways that you have been both intentionally and unintentionally dishonest. Please gently consider that to not tell others what you need, think, or feel, or to act as if you are perfect, hiding your vulnerabilities and struggles, is deceptive. It's unfair and inequitable.

Have you ever had a relationship with someone who is always doing great, who has no problems or needs? It's hard to feel close or connected to that person. Expressing sadness draws us closer to others. Otherwise, there is no way for others to know if they have hurt or offended you. They never get the chance to make things right. This lack of expression even makes me nervous in therapeutic relationships. I cannot know when clients are overwhelmed by an assignment unless they tell me. They may not tell me because they feel they must be "good" or strong enough to do whatever I ask, and I may never know that I am making things worse for them. It is ultimately up to all of us to know for ourselves, and then let others know, what is and what is not in our best interest.

Being honest with others carries some responsibility. Be sure to speak your truth to others in ways that are consistent with your long-term values and how you want to treat others. I have had clients who have told me that I don't care about them, and they hate me. They told me that they were just trying to be honest like I asked them to. I can handle and work with that as a therapist. But it does tend to alienate others and get in our way if we want or need any sort of relationship with them. Honesty is not an excuse for being unkind. It is possible to be honest in gentle, kind, and compassionate ways.

Act from Your Truth

Eating Disorder: "You made the wrong decision. If you had stayed at that job, you would be happy. Now you are miserable because you made a stupid decision. You're so stupid."

Truth: There is rarely such a thing as a perfect decision. Most decisions will have outcomes that we both like and dislike. We gather the facts, make the best decision we can, and get on with our lives. If the outcome is unacceptable, we make a decision to address that.

Though you are probably not ready to trust your decisions, it is important to keep practicing making the best ones you can, based on facts. The outcome of most decisions will have aspects that you both like and don't like. For instance, if you encounter a problem in a new job, you might not consider the possible negatives of having stayed at your old one. You might conclude that you would be happier, or at least less miserable, if you had not changed jobs. Do not use this feeling to beat yourself up for making a "bad" or "stupid" decision. Most decisions are reversible to some degree. So practice making the best decisions you can with the information you have, and remember that berating yourself if you dislike the outcome is not helpful. Making decisions is how we build the skill of making and learning to trust our decisions.

Another way to act from your truth is to back up verbal limits you set with others by knowing what you do or don't have control over, and acting within those limits. If you don't, you run the risk of feeling powerless, then running to your eating disorder and its illusions of control. That's exactly the place you are working so hard to stay away from. The next tool can help you find ways to set your limits with others and hold those limits with your actions, if necessary. Other people, often unaware of what is helpful or harmful in your journey toward recovery, may say and do things that leave you reeling and trigger intense eating-disorder thoughts and feelings.

 1) Make a list of all the triggering words you can imagine hearing from someone else. Examples: "I wish I could make myself throw up when I eat too much. I've tried but I can't." "Have you gained weight?" "You've lost some weight, you look good." "Just eat healthy food and don't buy junk food." 2) For each of these triggering words or phrases, write down what you might say, not say, do, or not do, when you hear them, then practice saying your responses out loud.

Examples:
- Sarcasm: "I can't tell you. It's classified information."
- Radical Genuineness: "It's a complex and difficult thing to have to go through."
- Education: "When you say, 'You look good,' my eating disorder twists it to mean that I'm fat."
- Statistics: "Diets don't work. Within five years, dieters gain back the weight they lost plus more."
- Fogging: "I'd prefer not to talk about that." (Continue same statement until they run out of steam.)
- Quick getaway: "Oh geez! I'm late. Gotta go!" (Briskly walk away.)

Always remember that just because someone asks you a question does not mean you are obligated to provide the information he or she is asking for. You have some control here. However, in the best interest of your recovery, it is to your advantage to teach those in your life what is helpful, not helpful, and harmful to say to you. You teach others through what you say, what you don't say, what you do, and what you don't do. Ultimately, it is up to us to coach others on how we need to be treated.

Use both your brain and your emotions. Use your voice. Use your actions. Take pride in uncovering your truths as you walk through this life. Hold your head high and speak your truth with conviction, kindness, and seriousness. Live your truths. Bring your actions into alignment with your values and goals. This is the blueprint not only for the structure of recovery from your eating disorder, but for your dream home . . . a life that is worth living.

Everyone has a guide on the inside.
And its name is not "eating disorder."
Its name is "Truth."

Today, I will embrace my authentic self.
Who I really am and what I have to say is
worth attention. I now give that attention
to myself by showing up for my life.

11.
Self-Care Is the New Beautiful

Deep Gratitude and a Final Good-bye

By Robyn

Six years ago, I stood on the other side of the world, where childhood memories rose to choke me with their finality, and good-byes that were not welcome came anyway.

My plump, pregnant hands attempted to take in the essence of my mother's limp body as they stroked the few parts of her not intruded upon by machinery. Her frail body lay dying as I stood beside her full of life, baby within kicking in time to my heartbeat, as hers was kept alive artificially. My hands fumbled around tubes and needles as I quietly cried with the awareness that my mum, the woman whom I depended upon and who was my everything, was about to leave this world, one short month before my first child would be born.

My mum saw me for three years in recovery. She saw me marry the man I had fallen for in a way that she had never witnessed in the past. She saw the connection of soul mates in us, and then she saw me pregnant, something she had never envisioned because of my illness. She saw her little girl's essence return, an essence that could create a bubble of laughter around her when she spoke. She saw me, the real me, and I thank God so much for those three years. I know now that I soothed my mum's soul by being in recovery. I know as a parent that the love we have for our children is unconditional and deeper than any other love one can experience. I know that my illness caused sleepless nights and the emotional torture of questioning what part she may have had in it. Parents always question their part, even though they can't save their children from eating disorders, for no one has that power. My mum let go of that guilt and deep sadness for her child in the last three years of her life. I am so grateful that I have that to look back on now.

One of the last conversations I had with my mum showed me that I had changed in my recovery. She was struggling to breathe as the lupus attacked her lungs and told her body that her organs were not her own. Again, on the other side of the world, on the phone—this time, I was able to be there for *her*. She was scared, and she told me so, an open dialogue I will treasure till my own death. "I am scared, Robbie." "Of course you are, Mum," I said softly. I remember being so conscious of needing to hear her, honor her truth, and love her to her death. We both knew she was dying. It was an unspoken thing that my mother conveyed to me with her thoughts. We had always had that connection. Even on the other side of the world, my mum knew when something was wrong with me. She would call me and say, "What's wrong Robbie-Lou?" I now experienced that with her, and I comforted *her*. One of the last things she said to me was, "Oh thank you, Robbie, you have made me feel so much better."

I am so grateful for recovery.

Nearly two weeks after arriving home from my mother's bedside, now thirty-six weeks along, I sat clad in old, plaid pajamas, the only item that provided my pregnant body comfort. Tim and I cuddled close on our sofa, with the TV acting as white noise. We weren't really watching anything; we were buying time until our life changed. Those last weeks of pregnancy had me nesting at home, making sure we had everything ready for our little soon-to-be Lilly, our own family. Then the phone rang. I knew it was my brother. It wasn't the "no-caller ID" that came up on the blinking phone screen that gave it away, but the air of freeness that lingered around our tiny Santa Monica apartment. I believe it was the freeness of my mother's soul leaving her physical pain behind. We felt that. That. We felt *that*.

"She's gone, Bub," my brother croaked.

I couldn't speak, as the long-awaited death was now absolute. I took a breath and held my stomach as my mind froze with the shock. I mumbled something to my brother, and as I hung up the phone, holding my arms around my baby's bulge, I screamed with a primal, wounded rawness. And then I screamed again. I screamed in the hope of catching my mum's spirit as she passed beyond us, out of this lifetime. How can I continue to live? I thought. She's gone. She is *gone*. I let out a scream again, this time for my unborn children.

You see, the truth was, I *could* live, however unbearable that reality felt. The universe made it so with a baby of my own to live for. Life is mysterious and magical and painful all in one. I am blessed that my mum lived nineteen additional years from the day the doctor told her to tell her family of her imminent death. I am indebted that I had her to teach me what being a women and a mommy meant. I take this with me now as I raise my own children. I am thankful that I hear her words, still, when I need advice; when I am still and so very quiet, I hear them. I am grateful that when she died, I became more of the woman I wanted to become through every step I took following my recovery. My mum was never again on the end of the phone, but her lessons were instilled deep within me. I learned to confide in myself, and I grew up because of it. I know she would be proud of me. I am grateful that she showed me what self-care looked like as she refused to give in to her illness. The measures she went to in order to care for herself now pave the way for me.

I am also grateful for my girls, who showed me the love my mum had for me. I understand that death is not something I should push myself toward for peace, but a sacredness beyond any mind's comprehension, one that is final. I am grateful that today I get to be present in a conversation after having eaten a meal; the meal has no power over me. Once eaten, it is over—period (just like it was meant to be). I am grateful that I understand now that I don't have any control over this world and the people and things in it; this responsibility and pressure to be in control is pointless and too heavy, anyway. I am grateful for the mystery in this life, and that even when I think I know; I often don't. I take comfort in this world being so much bigger than I ever imagined, and that I am but a blip on the radar—and most days, that is enough for me. I take pride in letting go and seeing life on life's terms. I am grateful that I have the confidence to walk through anything and be okay, for I have walked through death, bankruptcy, an eating disorder, and depression. None have killed me; and yes, they have made me stronger. I have shut the door on my illness because it has no place or need in my life today. Today I walk through life, not fearless, not perfect, not knowing what is around the corner, full of fault . . . but still okay.

◆ ◆ ◆

Now that I know unequivocally that I can eat whatever I want when I am hungry and stop when I am full, I have also discovered how the actual foods make me feel. This is what Espra and I call the Self-Care Approach to eating in our Nutritional Healing: A Three-Tier Approach™. I know that eating a pastry full of sugar for breakfast makes me tired by noon. I know that I need carbohydrates to sleep well. For me, too much time without food makes me shaky and irritable (the list goes on); it is a reminder that I am off-track. I have also discovered that the moment I consider "cutting back" on foods I love, I actually want to eat them more. I cannot diet, for with every diet a binge is lurking. Unfortunately, there are a lot of wages that are paid via the diet industry, so I need to have discernment for myself. Dieting for me is craziness. It means that I am out of touch with my body's mind and my emotional well-being. Emotional well-being, for me, is vital to my recovery.

I have "broken glasses" (body dysmorphia), sometimes, still. When I get emotional or rundown and don't feel good about a situation I tend to look in the mirror and see a large lady staring back at me. Now, in recovery I don't take it so seriously. My body no longer owns my definition of self. Today, I am able to shift my perception of self without self-destruction, and repair my glasses so that I can see my body more accurately.

I would not take back my process of food discovery and recovery, ever. I truly mean this. I have learned so much about myself through my food choices that now provide me with a strong foundation for my fully recovered life. But it wasn't enough not to be body obsessed anymore and to be able to eat whatever I wanted; I also craved optimum health. You know the kind of thing "normal" people speak about and we took to mean another tactic to lose weight? It really exists. Optimum health is discovering what makes you feel your best and being capable of honoring it. I now cherish my life and my ever-growing zest for it, and want to be my best self in it.

There is a reason why this chapter is here at the end of the book and not at the beginning: maybe you feel like I once did. I could not have been truthful and curious about my body in a way that promotes optimum health when I was beginning recovery. My mind was not there yet. My body had lost contact with my mind years ago, and I needed to reconnect them first. I was able to via the Structured Approach, and I strengthened the relationship via the Mindful Approach. A while back I was involved in a discussion with two women of my extended family about one of their concepts of "good" and "bad" food. When one of the women said, "Robyn *loves* her food. With the amount she eats, she should be the size of a house." The other lady cringed, as I think she may have taken this comment to be careless, even hurtful, but I knew it was not really about trying to criticize me, nor was she commenting on *my* food intake as it *really* was. Like most of us, she has been taught our cultural "norm." You see, I think she may have been complimenting me. By saying that it was due to my genes that I was not fat, she was insinuating that I was a "lucky" woman who had dodged the bullet of having to watch every morsel that enters my mouth. The truth? She has been deceived by our society to believe that dieting is the answer to optimal health. Like most of us, she has been fed the lies instead of the truth of diets and their danger to bring us further away from our body's intelligence and make us feel emotionally overwhelmed in the process. My body structure was created from my gene pool, yes, but I also follow a general rule: If I am hungry and the food that is available to me is something my body wants, I eat it. Sometimes it is not what I want, but I have to eat something because my body is asking for it, so I make do and eat anyway. If I am not hungry, I don't eat. I no longer feel like "I have to eat it because tomorrow I can't." It's that simple, really. I am far from what my extended family member might call a "big eater," but yes, I do love my food. Dieting has become a part of our culture, but I don't have to buy into it or be a part of it. This is part of my self-care today.

To me, self-care is knowing the things that make me feel good about myself, that help me speak my truth and support my needs as an individual, and then acting on them to best honor myself. Self-care in all it represents is my new definition of beautiful. It's so much more fulfilling than the media's definition—so much more inspiring, liberating, and obtainable.

At this stage of my recovery, it is also about optimum health. Ten years into it, I still have to remind myself about my responsibility to self-care. I understand that my body needs a certain amount of exercise, protein, sleep, hydration, fun, laughter, "me" time, quiet time, "Mommy, Lilly, and Chloe" time, "no computer" time, "Tim and Robyn" time, and good ol' "chit-chat with my best friend, Andi" time. Sometimes I still choose to have food that I have discovered I am sensitive to. But it's a conscious choice that is not laden with guilt or shame. I sense that, like everything, when I've had enough of the energy zaps I will let go of it organically. I try to encourage my little girls to eat this way too. There is no "good" or "bad" food in our house, just "energy" food and "fun" food. Our home has many "fun" foods within it that I do not think twice about today, for food has no power here anymore.

I know that self-care is in my pauses, in my willingness to give up the illusion of control. It is in being present, in being able to laugh at myself; it is in pursuing my dreams and loving to the best of my ability. I know this about me because *I now know me.*

How to Appreciate Something as a Path to Loving It

By Espra

What Does Self-Care Mean to You?

Eating Disorder: "It means, 'Stop eating so much, you pig.'"

Truth: Self-care is a practice, and it is a wide path that shifts with the moment, circumstance, and life. Self-compassion is the middle path, somewhere between self-indulgence and self-deprivation.

Society, the media, and those around us give conflicting messages about self-care. Self-sacrifice is often touted as a quality of a "good" person, while self-care can be considered self-indulgent. Relying on others to decide what self-care means for you can leave you confused and vulnerable. That's when you risk buying into the eating disorder's self-deprivation mindset regarding food and self-care in general. You are then at risk of restricting yourself to only certain foods or amounts, while the eating disorder says you are using self-care and "healthy eating."

When you get to this stage in your recovery, you can more readily tune in and respect the quiet voice inside you that knows depriving and punishing yourself does not create a life worth living. Each of us must identify where and how it is helpful to nurture and reward ourselves as part of our individual path of self-care. The challenge is to walk your personal path of self-care, notice when you stray to either side, then move back to it and just begin again. Remember, different standards do not apply to you just because you are "unworthy," "undeserving," or different than everyone else in any other way (that's eating-disorder thinking).

From Perfection and Guilt to Curious and Proud

Eating Disorder: "Once you're perfect, you can feel good about yourself. Self-compassion is an excuse for self-indulgence and laziness.

Permission to do or be anything less than perfect opens the door to becoming the big, fat slob you deserve to be."

Truth: Believing these lies will pretty much guarantee that you remain loyal to the eating disorder. Breaking free requires doing the *opposite* of what the eating disorder is telling you to do or, in the words of my clients, "faking it till you make it."

Focusing on making yourself perfect leads you toward feeling guilty and miserable, not happy. As you move away from self-deprivation and perfectionism toward self-care, prepare for your eating-disorder thoughts to deliver guilt and shame. The eating disorder thrives on your self-deprivation, telling you how bad you are and helping you always remember it. Eating disorders insist that depriving, judging, and punishing yourself are the only ways to keep you motivated to do what you are "supposed to do."

If you feel like you don't deserve to relax for ten minutes, relax anyway, because that quiet inner voice beneath the eating disorder's chatter knows it is helpful for you. Talk back, insisting that a life of meaning and quality is built upon developing pride in acting in congruence with your authentic self, not your rigid and inflexible self. If you are tired, go to bed earlier. If relaxing in bed is how you avoid your life, then get out of bed more often. Each moment brings a new chance for you to either batter yourself with guilt about your imperfections or orient yourself back toward the path of self-care. Beginning again means focusing your mind on being curious about both the pleasant and the scary things that lie beyond your bed, instead of punishing yourself for having been there in the first place. As you replace your self-deprivation rituals with intuitive and authentic actions, you begin living from authentic power and diminishing the power of the eating disorder. Everything, initially, will feel like self-indulgence. Work hard to mold your thinking from guilt and obsession with perfection at any cost, into curiosity and the kind of pride each of us finds in self-respect.

Your Body, Acceptance, and Appreciation

Eating Disorder: "Are you joking? Now they're trying to convince you that you're hallucinating when you see your own fat body."

Truth: Individuals who suffer with eating disorders are at high risk of having "broken glasses," which cause them to see their body as 25 percent, 30 percent, or as much as double its actual size or more.

Robyn understood and worked to accept that a symptom of her eating disorder was that she literally saw the size and shape of her body as completely different than its actual size or shape.

In the case of eating disorders, even weight loss does not cause the body to appear small enough to decrease the resulting disgust. Eating-disorder professionals refer to this body image distortion as "body dysmorphia." My clients call body image distortion things like, "the eating disorder messing with your head."

Regardless of how you personally refer to these "broken glasses," you are at high risk of having a distorted body image as a symptom of your eating disorder. The resulting self-consciousness and obsessive preoccupation with your body are consuming to the point that even conversations and activities can become miserable and seemingly impossible. Feigning interest while being distracted by checking and hiding your body's flaws is exhausting, and many with eating disorders avoid people and activities as much as possible.

Your perception of your body may have been inaccurate before your eating disorder started, but the eating disorder makes it worse. To compound the problem, another characteristic of eating disorders is placing a greater emphasis on the shape or size of your body than on other aspects of yourself as the means of determining your personal value and worth. You are in quite a fix. You are at risk of seeing your body as larger than it actually is, and what you see in the mirror defines you as worthless and disgusting. To say that the eating disorder has set you up to be miserable is an understatement.

Not yet satisfied, as usual, the eating disorder carries on to convince you that the rest of the world also notices, stares, and feels disgusted by your body. This is another lie. Yes, some people do judge our bodies and other things they dislike about us because some people are just that way and our culture encourages it. It is their own need to compare and judge who comes out as "better" or "worse" than themselves, and it has no more to do with your worth than your comparisons have to do with theirs. But the ways in which others judge you are rarely as horrific as your eating disorder would have you believe or as those assaults the eating disorder personally delivers to you. Talk back: How many people have you observed running out of the room and gagging immediately after you walk in? Others tend to be put off more by someone who's preoccupied with their own body than the size of that person's body. When you are preoccupied with comparing bodies, looking at your reflection, and adjusting your body and clothes, people can lose interest in being around you. It is obvious that your focus is elsewhere, and they feel ignored. Logical conclusion: It is more likely that your behaviors, rather than your appearance, make others feel awkward and uncomfortable around you. Perhaps it's the eating disorder, not your body that is undesirable to others. Think about this and talk back!

Because you see your body with your own two eyes (though your vision is probably distorted), others cannot convince you that they view your body very differently than you do. Additionally, you might feel frustrated when they tell you so. Recovery means educating yourself about your broken glasses, then constantly reminding yourself that body dysmorphia is a symptom of eating disorders, yours included. Work with your therapist and other resources to find concrete ways to challenge your view of your body rather than relying on broken glasses. Questioning your perception of the size and shape of your body is frightening but important. Ironically, improving self-esteem, rather than losing weight, is the treatment for body dysmorphia. Broken glasses can be mended as you build gratitude, appreciation, and curiosity for how your body works and what it can do.

Write a list of things you can do because you have a body. Review and appreciate these things once or more each day.

Examples: Hug someone, look at the ocean, feel the sun on my face, pet my dog, listen to music, walk in nature, play a sport, or fly a kite.

Discover for yourself how appreciating the body you have, not pushing to make it a certain way, is the key to happiness. You may never love your body, and, honestly, few people do. The key to creating a life worth living is getting curious about your body and the miracle of it. When you teach yourself to appreciate the ways your body helps you live a meaningful life and use your body to do just that, you break free from having to rely on your appearance to measure your worth. You accept the body you have, appreciate what it can do for you, and love it for showing up for you.

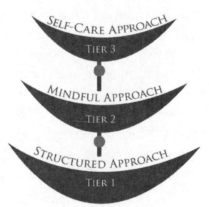

NUTRITIONAL HEALING: A 3-TIER APPROACH™

Tier Three: The Self-Care Approach to Eating

Eating Disorder: "That's easy. Self-care means eating healthy. Otherwise you'll get fat and have health problems."

Truth: The research is clear. Health problems that have traditionally been blamed on "weighing too much" are more often related to imbalance in lifestyle than weight itself. So move over, eating disorder, we don't have time for your trash. We have work to do.

Our Self-Care Approach to eating considers structure, your preferences, and moves beyond them to target your body's chemical and biological idiosyncrasies as well as its ever-changing needs. You are ready for the Self-Care Approach when your emotions or worries related to food no longer drive your choices. For the most part, fear is replaced by faith in your body and your ability to care for it in your human, imperfect, evolving, and curious way.

The Self-Care Approach is eating for optimum health. The Self-Care Approach is both mindful and structured eating, not self-depriving or rigid eating. You must be well practiced in both the Structured Approach and the Mindful Approach to eating before you attempt the Self-Care Approach. We suggest at least a year of practicing the Structured Approach and at least another year practicing the Mindful Approach before you consider incorporating the Self-Care Approach. It is crucial not to rush or skip the first two stages, as they decrease fears of food and making food choices to build self-trust, which is the essence of what you will ultimately need to quiet the eating disorder. The Self-Care Approach is the next step, as it helps you tune in to your body's responses to food over time. You may discover relationships between things like food types, amounts; times of the day, month, and year; and how they affect your body. This helps you shift (not restrict) what you eat and when you eat it to fit your needs at the time.

Note: We suggest at least a year of practicing the Structured Approach and at least another year practicing the Mindful Approach before you consider incorporating the Self-Care Approach.

With the Self-Care Approach, you loosely use structure with times of day and a range of foods. You know you like some foods more than others; you accept that you can eat what you want without guilt; and now you will begin to discover how different foods give your body advantages or disadvantages that others do not. Within the Self-Care Approach you become curious about how foods affect your well-being, and can begin to make choices in eating the foods that make you feel good in the big picture, as opposed to only eating the foods that immediately zap your energy, or do so on the heels of a quick rush.

Within the Structured Approach you can start to listen beyond your desires for certain foods, when your body becomes hungry. For example: If you need energy, attend to your body's messages about foods that give you energy, immediate and/or long-lasting. The antithesis of self-care is using certain foods, like caffeine or sugar, as "drugs" to give you a quick buzz of energy. *And* self-care for you might mean having caffeinated drinks and sweet or "carb-filled" foods when they sound good, or might give you a quick, fleeting energy surge, while being mindful that it is a choice rather than a thoughtless habit or pattern.

The Self-Care Approach is about recognizing what foods do for and to you. It's about using your nutrition to provide you with optimal physical, mental, and emotional functioning and wellness (according to your body's responses, not eating-disorder reactions). Optimal physical functioning can be measured by things like energy that lasts longer than otherwise, increased strength, even mood and emotional responses, clearer thinking, and your body feeling at ease. For example, I often crave ice cream, convinced it's what my body wants, when I haven't eaten in the past four to five hours—when anyone would likely be experiencing low sugar levels. In those cases, I try to honor my desire for sweet, cold, and creamy, but at the same time, I am mindful of how my body may respond. I recognize that if I go for the ice cream in the middle of my work day, a time where I need more lasting energy, the outcome will most likely not benefit my productivity. I know I will be less likely to think clearly, irritable, shaky, and have less mental and physical energy. Using the Self-Care Approach I am able to consider my outcomes and make my choices accordingly. Self-care eating is about being able to make these choices without the eating disorder nudging or interfering. Instead of ice cream, I may decide to go for yogurt or anything else that provides more energy yet honors my body's desire for a sweet, cold, and creamy texture.

Often, abstinence from foods that you like, but that leave your body functioning below its optimal level, is unnecessary. That decision needs to be made between you and your body, and if necessary, your healthcare provider. Warning: The eating disorder is not a member of your healthcare team.

You find true freedom from the eating disorder as you move from its directives of "healthy" or "what you deserve" to your own body's wisdom of true nutritional self-care. Your blueprint for nutritional recovery must include the full repertoire of nutritional responses in life. Whether you are in a situation where you have many or only a few food options, you use what is available to refuel your body when needed. The eating disorder would have you either run your tank dry, waiting for the "perfect" fuel source, or indiscriminately fueling up, possibly overflowing your tank with little deliberate preparation. The Self-Care Approach is eating to keep your body, brain, and chemistry working optimally throughout the day. Using your Structured Approach skills, you "top off" every four or five hours to keep your body at an even level. Using your Mindful Approach, you are less afraid to top off with more food if you are hungry and less if you are not. You choose what your body wants from the range of food options available, and you use what is available when needed. After practicing the Structured Approach sufficiently, it becomes a natural, safe place. You own your Structured Approach; it is yours; it never fails and never goes away, as long as you are willing to go back to it when necessary. Robyn says that the foundation of her Structured Approach is now an ingrained part of her that she naturally falls back upon. When she is sick and her appetite decreases, Robyn knows that her Structured Approach is part of her way back and says, "It's quite brilliant, really, to have the solution within myself." Can you see how the Structured Approach *is* the Self-Care Approach? As long as you remember this, your body's mind will be capable of returning you to the Mindful Approach then the Self-Care Approach.

Watch your physical responses to the foods you eat for one day. Keep track of what you notice is happening with your body, mind, and mood with respect to the foods you eat and when you eat them. Notice how long after you've eaten certain foods your body begins responding with the outcomes you listed. Ask yourself after eating a particular food how your body responds. Examples: Does your body respond with a quick rush? Improved mental clarity? Do you feel less sluggish? Irritable? Do you have more energy or endurance? Does your energy crash? Are you shaky, tired, washed out, weak?

After you gather this information about your body's responses to certain foods, you are positioned to experiment, and the next time you are hungry make a conscious choice that may result in a more desirable physical outcome. You are not locked into always making choices this way. In fact, sometimes you won't, and you alone can choose when it is necessary and when it is not. This is choice. This is power.

For example: When I'm taking a long hike and stop for a break, I know that I need to have a little bit of candy, salty food, and jerky. The salt protects my electrolytes, the sugar gives me immediate energy to resume hiking, and the protein brings a delayed, longer-lasting energy for my body to use after the energy from sugar is spent. However, if I am sitting at a desk all day doing research, I may not make the same food choices.

• •

If the eating disorder is poking you and whispering, "Hey don't forget about 'good,' 'bad,' 'diet' or 'comfort' foods," don't panic. It's okay; you've come a long way. Just notice that you are off track and may feel a little unsafe. If this is the case, bring your mind back to a recovery mindset, your wise mind, and go back to the Mindful Approach or if necessary the Structured Approach to eating until you have regained your physical and mental stability with food. At the end of the day, if you are working on this phase and your intuitive sense is raising a red flag, don't worry, just go back and try this phase again when it feels right.

Wake Up and Show Up

Eating Disorder: "Yes, why don't you wake up their way, and see what shows up . . . on your thighs."

Truth: Can you now begin to move beyond the eating disorder's focus only on your body as a way to show up in life? There is no guarantee that your body will or won't change from improved self-care, but I am convinced that your life will change for the better.

As you learn to listen to your body, your heart and your mind take their places in the balance of your life. As you express your true desires and live your life based on what is in the best interest of your mind and body, the voice of the eating disorder begins to have less power over you. You will find its chatter less believable, your ability to challenge it increases, and the percentage of your day that it talks and your behaviors obey it decrease.

As your head clears and your behavior is not consumed by the eating disorder, you become able to look around you and see outside of yourself. You are opening your eyes and taking in information from your environment, versus your heart or head exclusively. You wake up to your world. You wake up to life.

Now your recovery, instead of your eating disorder, is starting to take on a life of its own. Now you can sincerely listen, hear without distraction, see, and respond to your life. Your relationships deepen and become more meaningful . . . not because you have created a perfect body, but because you are showing up. You are showing true compassion instead of constantly comparing yourself to others. You are finding things to discuss other than food, exercise, and _____ (fill in the blank). People are responding to you because you have interesting things to say. When you live in a place of self-care, you do not eat perfectly; you eat imperfectly while showing up (for yourself and others) and expressing yourself in a perfectly imperfect way. You are perfectly human, and you immerse yourself in the enduring things that matter to you most in the context of your long-term goals and values. When you do this, you are filling yourself with your authentic power. Living in this way is not an illusion, it's living!

Playing it safe is like poking yourself in the eye.
Ultimately you lose sight of all
the magic around you.

*Today, I will allow myself to take
part in the world around me.
Life is worth my attention. I am worth the world!*

12.

Make Recovery Worth It

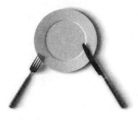

Dreams and Bottom Drums

By Robyn

Although recovery has long been entrenched in my bones and my thought process naturally steers toward it, I am sometimes still fascinated by the odd sensation of looking back at my behavior during my eating disorder and being unable to grasp what kept me in a life near death for so many years. I still remember the pain I inflicted on those who loved me while in my illness, and although the guilt and shame sometimes still stings, I have learned that it serves no one to stay stuck in pain. I now work hard to reach out to those people with the hand of the *real* me, and with that, gently encourage myself to move forward.

Recovery is something palpable and tangible, just as my fear was when driven by my eating disorder. Only now it's sensational in a positive way, not a punch-in-the-gut kind of way. It is because of this change that I want to share recovery with you. Because if you had told me ten years ago that I could feel the way I do today, I would have called you a liar. I would have told you that you don't know me or my body; therefore, you couldn't possibly tell me that I could do it. If you knew me better, you would understand. Like I said before, I am part European. I am prone to curvy hips, lady mustaches, and a mix of a deep, dark depression that, if exposed, might kill me. "So let me be," I would have warned you, with a look in my eyes that would distance you in a heartbeat. *Let me be.* I am destined to walk this life chained to my fateful eating disorder, worthless, alone, and hopeless. But now I sit here and I am telling you that you too can feel recovery! I don't care what you say is different about you. Eating disorders do not discriminate. We are the same, and you too can be free from it and the underlying issues that may hide beneath it, if you want to be.

One of the questions I have asked myself is, "What does recovery mean to me?" Recovery, for me, means showing up for myself and others. Recovery means being able to be present. It means accepting imperfections and life on life's terms. It means feeling my feelings, and with that, experiencing real pain, real discomfort, real happiness, laughter, hope, and . . . me. Recovery means experiencing the sensation of running, but standing still anyway. It means laughing at myself sometimes. It means being open to the magic of our glorious and sometimes scary world. I reflect on this to remind myself of what I can do now that I could not do when my life was dictated by body image and eating-disorder anguish. When I get quiet and find one thing that recovery means to me, other gifts, other things that I can do in recovery come flooding in on me, until a sense of gratitude permeates my being.

Recovery does not mean that life will, from now on, be perfect. There simply isn't such a thing. Being perfect or striving for it is not what my recovery is about; it's the complete opposite actually. The pursuit of perfection brings with it similar sensations to that of an eating disorder. I run from it like a burning building. Albeit, sometimes I still have to feel the burn of the flame before I decide to run, but I do end up running. Today I say no to eating disorder and no to perfection. Recovery does not mean that I no longer have to work on myself. I no longer hide from the fact that there are underlying issues such as trauma, depression, anxiety, low self-esteem, and other difficulties that I need to trudge through as part of my recovery, as part of life. The things that led me to hide from myself and my life are now the things I face. My need to "be someone," my desire to control my family's lives so that I do not have to worry about them, or the chronic state of busyness I get trapped in all have to be recognized and balanced. After all, these are the things that brought me to my eating disorder in the first place.

The real payoffs for me, however, are the little things that make it all worth it, like when I hear the outside noise of the birds getting on with their morning as they sit on the stripped branches of winter singing to all who will listen. Or when out of the blue, I feel uncomfortable and I can check in with myself, without the noise and violence of the eating disorder, and discover what is really going on. This makes recovery worth it for me. When I can feel bored, impatient, and frustrated without having to look in the fridge or the mirror, but instead, call a friend, focus on a task that requires attention, or just sit with my feelings. This makes recovery worth it for me. And when my little girls comment on the shape of my bottom and pat it like a drum, and I can shake it off without feeling that I have failed—this peace and ease with who I am makes recovery, and indeed life, worth it.

It is not that life is magical *all* of the time. I would be steering you wrong if I were to say that life is always grand and that all I have in my life is perfect. Sometimes I still feel larger than I am, and sometimes life feels messy. I know these moments well. I understand now that when I feel vulnerable my body feels larger than it actually is. The difference today is I don't take those feelings to heart. I simply take action—action that centers me. I go back to basics, and I nurture myself in a way that makes me feel good about myself, not a way that punishes me for feeling imperfect.

In recovery I can be a part of a solution and a freedom and a peace that are just waiting for me to walk into and own. Life is fleeting. As I remind myself how I want to live it today, I know that I have choices. I know that I am all of the power I gave the eating disorder; I am me, and I am enough. I feel my feelings, and sometimes they still feel unbearable. But now I know that they will pass, and I will feel free from them again soon if I do not judge them. Sometimes too I still feel "less than," especially when I create expectations for myself that are not appropriate for my skills or circumstances. That's okay. Because I know how courageous I can be and how, now that I am in recovery, I can follow my dreams and know that everything that I am doing is enough. Doing my best is enough. I know that I don't and will never have all the answers in life, nor do I know what will come of my efforts. But putting my efforts into my dreams provides me with self-worth and self-esteem, because I am finally doing everything I always wanted. I define my own worth, dreams, truth, power, and beauty.

You see, this is *my* life. I can make it a playground or a prison. It is my choice. It is my day.

Just as it is yours!

Create Your Own Drums

By Espra

Know What Recovery Means

Eating Disorder: "You can eat, and you can stop getting rid of calories. You can also have a miserable life, because that's how recovery will be."
Truth: A life of value, quality, and meaning grows from saying no to the eating disorder.

Most of my clients have been afraid that recovery would mean a lifetime of abstaining from eating-disorder behaviors despite the constant barrage of eating-disorder thoughts and feelings of misery. Although it seems impossible to live without eating-disorder behaviors and with less misery, both are possible. In fact, the less you practice eating-disorder behaviors, the more the chatter backs off. But do not expect the eating disorder's chatter and lies to completely die out right away. It takes time for the chatter to diminish, so please don't give up when you become frustrated that it does not back off as quickly as it "should." The eating disorder's assaults will actually increase initially, known in psychology as an "extinction burst," before it begins to back down. Then, even as it retreats, it will return to batter you in waves. But if you pay careful attention, you will probably be able to observe that its assaults, gradually and with time, decrease in intensity, frequency, and/or duration. I wish I created this phenomenon because then I could change it. The best I can do is explain how the eating disorder will behave as you challenge it. So be sure to acknowledge that you are changing.

Since no one in their right mind would pursue recovery without real reasons to do so, keep the reasons you are seeking recovery alive in your mind by frequently referring back to the tools you have used throughout this book. You may add to or alter the tools as you work with them over time. Just make sure you do so from a logical perspective, rather than basing them on fears prompted by the eating disorder's emotional appeals. You may be extremely uncomfortable in the earlier parts of recovery, as new ways of interacting with the eating disorder and your world throw you out of the status quo and into a sort of chaos. For a while, the new ways will not feel comfortable, so you may go back to habitual patterns. But soon the old, familiar patterns will become less comfortable, leaving you feeling like neither your new behaviors nor your old ones fit. Stay with the discomfort, and the new ways will become new patterns and habits; they will become the new status quo.

No matter what your eating disorder may tell you, a full and complete recovery is attainable, not only for others, but also for you.

Research shows that a complete recovery from eating disorders is possible. My mentors teach that individuals can and do make a full recovery from eating disorders. Many of my clients have proven to themselves and to me that recovery is possible. Like Robyn, you will become less dependent on the eating disorder's illusions that being "skinny," "perfect," or sick is the only way to get your needs met. You will become more capable as you cultivate the skills to meet your needs in ways that are more skillful and effective and less destructive to yourself and those around you. No matter what your eating disorder may tell you, a full and complete recovery is attainable, not only for others, but also for you.

Shortly after Robyn heard that she should be as big as a house due to what she eats, Robyn called me. When Robyn told me what happened, my words hit no speed bumps before rushing out to ask what she thought and felt about those words. I wondered if she had flashes of guilt or shame, and if those brought up eating-disorder thoughts or urges to restrict or purge. Robyn told me that she did notice a thought: "With the amount that I eat, I should be exactly the size that I am, thank you very much." She walked away from that situation without contempt for herself or her body, but with sadness for what society so convincingly teaches us—that self-deprivation and "self-control" is the only way to have a body that is "good enough" to make the person "good enough." I was already clear, but if there was any doubt remaining, I was certain at that moment that Robyn had fully recovered from her eating disorder.

Food, body, and thoughts of inadequacy still show up among the other irritating thoughts we all occasionally have. The difference is that now they won't grab your attention, emotions, or behavior in the same way . . . and they certainly won't run your life. Society will not stop trying to impose its rules on you about how your body must look a certain way and be forced into an unrealistic mold to be good enough. As you identify those things of higher meaning and value in your life, you are no longer at the mercy of the eating disorder's illusions. You will notice the thoughts of inadequacy and keep right on doing whatever you are doing in that moment. You will keep right on living your life, striving to immerse yourself in the preciousness of the very moment you are in—before the moment is lost forever.

Know What "Worth It" Means

Eating Disorder: "The only way you can be happy without me is to be happy being fat."
Truth: The only way to be happy without the eating disorder is to be willing to be without the eating disorder.

By now you know that the eating disorder has insane expectations about perfect bodies and controlling eating. You know the eating disorder moves the finish line as soon as you cross it, insisting that its prior goal is no longer good enough, and you have to do even more and be better. It can move that bar until death do you part.

Both joy and suffering are parts of all of our lives. Happiness is a fleeting state that does not permanently hang around with us. What makes recovery worthwhile is your ability to live a life that aligns with your long-term goals and values. It is a sort of peace and relaxing into your life. Recovery is worth it when you begin to have faith in your ability to cope with anger, fear, sadness, guilt, shame, happiness, love, and *all* emotions without the need to do anything but coexist with them. Recovery is worth it when you fully experience your life.

Look back through the tools you have created as you have used this book and find the ones that reference values, interests, passions, and goals. Choose just one of your authentic values, interests, passions, or goals as a starting place for your next step. List all of the steps you would have to take to make that particular goal real for you. If you feel overwhelmed after listing the steps, go back and insert smaller steps in between the larger ones. All steps are possible when you make them small enough.

• •

Play. Enjoy. It's Your Life!

Eating Disorder: "Playing is a waste of time. You need to do things that are meaningful and worthwhile."

Truth: That which is meaningful and worthwhile can only be defined by you and can only be defined based on your core values and passions.

Planning pleasant things to do, big and small, doing them, and fully immersing yourself in them is part of the therapeutic treatment for shame and depression. Even if you are not enjoying yourself, act like you are anyway. This is not dishonesty; it is part of the emotional skill to decrease shame and sadness and depression. Besides, what possible benefit could come from sulking or distracting your way through a positive event anyway? Act interested and happy and, in the best case scenario, you and those around you just might enjoy the experience. Worst case scenario: it will go by faster if you are immersed in it, and you can decide not to try that experience again.

Take a piece of paper and make five columns. Down the left side, write the days of the week, with each day below the previous one, until you have listed all seven days of the week. To the right of each day, write one pleasant event (leave out the "shoulds" and "should nots") that you can plan to do that day. Then engage in a pleasant activity at least once per day. You might use the activity that you planned or you might do a different one. It doesn't really matter because the point is for you to engage in a pleasant activity. After you have done the activity, list what you did and whether or not you notice a decrease in any difficult moods you may have been experiencing before the event. The last column is for writing anything you noticed about yourself or the event as you attempted to show up with your body, mind, and heart present.

• •

Learning to be with others in the absence of the eating disorder's distorted thinking, talk, and behavior is yet another challenge and gift of recovery. As you show up physically, intellectually, and emotionally with other people, you identify those with whom you feel a sense of connection, trust, respect, and safety. The illusion that safety lies only in being loyal to the eating disorder grows fuzzy as you see glimpses of safety without it. The connection now begins between you and these caring others, as opposed to the isolation you experienced while at the mercy of your illness. You are able to receive the gifts others bring to you, sort through what you do and do not want to accept, then truly give the gifts of your soul that endure beyond calories, food, and clothing size.

Following Your Dreams
Eating Disorder: "But, but . . . "
Truth: That's right.

Recovery is worth it when you have an idea of your passions, values, dreams, and goals and you attend to them regularly, like tending a garden. As you sow your thoughts and actions, which are meant to make a long-lasting contribution to yourself and the life you have chosen to create, balanced emotions and healthy habits will blossom into maturity. Your garden will continue to need regular work and attention, but without the burden of seeking perfection every waking moment. Then, one day, you see evidence that you are reaping the ultimate harvest—a life that feels worth living. And it all becomes possible as *you* see and *you* acknowledge the eating disorder as the serious and real threat that it is to your life. It is like a devastating infestation of weeds that must be attended to. As you vigilantly challenge the eating disorder, you remove pieces of it from your life by the roots, like pulling one noxious weed at a time. Its ability to regenerate diminishes, then halts. You must always pay attention for evidence that the eating disorder is returning so you can quickly challenge the devastating threats it will pose if it is allowed to propagate. It is important to cultivate and replant periodically, as conditions change. But one thing does not change: you are sowing the seeds that, when put all together, will bear more and more of what you ultimately desire over time.

> **"Sew a thought and reap an act.**
> **Sew an act and reap a habit.**
> **Sew a habit and reap a lifetime.**
> **Sew a lifetime and reap a destiny."**
> **—Anonymous**

Stay awake and attentive. Recovery is a process of losing your way, noticing when you do, and, without self-punishment or denigration, getting right back on the path that takes you toward your authentic source of power. It is impossible for you to perfectly follow the path of living your dreams, values, and goals because you are human. Just don't quit. Do your best to keep your eyes on the path that takes you where you want to go. You deserve a life that feels worth living. You are strong enough to get there, and it is fully possible for you.

Stabilize your food in order to stabilize your body. Respect the reality: your body needs nutritional fuel and care. Then create peace with your body and food by cultivating peace with yourself. Practice mindful eating, and self-care in eating and in your life. Use your authentic power to challenge the eating disorder's illusions of power, over and over again. Don't try to recover alone and don't give up. Perfection is an illusion, and no amount of manipulating your body and spirit will change that. Trust and faith are all you have to go on for now. The only way to see and touch the gifts that await you is to gather your faith, take a deep breath, close your eyes, and jump in. Recovery is available to you . . . if you want it.

Breaking through the mountain—
rubble hitting, hurting, shocking
my head, my body, my spirit.
I want to give up.
Yet I want to live.

I can turn back,
but when I look forward
I can see something.
I am not sure what it is.
But I know there is something.

With a deep breath
I move one foot
in front of the other.
Not with resistance.
It is with trust
and the tools I have found
along the way.

Something—
happiness, I think . . .
is waiting for me on the other side.

*To all of you seeking recovery, you
are well on your way now.*

Resources

Skills Resources

Mindfulness Skills

Resources for learning about and practicing mindfulness skills can be found in a number of places, including Eastern mindfulness traditions like meditation and yoga. There are many apps for phones and YouTube videos with instructions and assistance for learning deep breathing, paced breathing, and progressive muscle relaxation. Although many great resources can be found here, it can be difficult to know which are consistent with evidence-based ways of using the skills and which are not. For that reason, it is most safe to refer to the other resources I provide as well, so you can tell the difference.

Deep Breathing

How to take a deep breath: First, you must uncurl your body. Our bodies were created with a miraculous involuntary response that makes our breathing stop or become shallow and causes us to curl up or *fold* when we are under the threat of a physical attack. For this reason, when you perceive a threat but are not in *physical* danger, you have to override your body's automatic responses and get air in so your body and brain can work again.

Exhale as fully and deeply as you can. Then inhale as slowly and fully as you comfortably can. Next exhale a little longer and deepen your inhalation as well. Repeat this step, while trying to lengthen the exhalation and inhalation. Try experimenting with this until you find a way to take longer and fuller breaths. Then time yourself and count your breaths for one minute. The goal is to continually lengthen the breath over a period of two to five minutes. Ten or fewer deep breaths per minute is considered a nice rate. Note to perfectionists: fewer than five breaths per minute can put your body into another kind of physiological stress, which will make things worse.

Experiment when you are not feeling highly emotional. First, put your body into a scared or anxious posture. Curl and hunch your shoulders forward and down toward your toes; suck in and tighten your stomach and chest muscles; pull your knees up toward your stomach; tuck your head down with your chin against your chest; and clench your arms together across your stomach, chest, or around your knees. Then, while holding this posture, take two or three good deep breaths. How well does it work? Now uncurl your body by pulling your head up and back, eyes up and forward, arms down, shoulders back as if you are pushing your shoulder blades together, chest out, spine straight, legs down, and feet on the floor. Then take two to three deep breaths. Do you notice a difference?

After you uncurl your body, imagine that you have several candles in front of you that you are trying to blow out. Notice that we do not suck or inhale out candles. We blow out candles. That is because our bodies have stronger muscles to push air out than to take air in, another brilliant mechanism designed to help you survive by pushing out obstacles that are blocking your airway. You can learn to use this for your benefit. Start breathing by pushing in on your upper belly to push air out as if you are blowing out candles. Then relax your chest and stomach, without working to inhale, and let your body naturally take air back in. On the next breath out, see if you can add two extra puffs, then relax and let your body naturally take in a long, deep, full breath. After three to five of these, people are usually able to decrease their panic and relax their body just enough to begin some focused work on regulating their breathing. Don't continue this style of breathing beyond one or two minutes or you might start feeling dizzy or lightheaded.

Paced Breathing

Instructions: Taking about one step per second, exhale as you walk six steps, pause for one step, and inhale as you walk four steps. Watch the seconds on a clock or timer as you breathe out for six seconds, pause for one second, and breathe in for four seconds. Find a favorite paced breathing video and audio guide on YouTube. Download one of the many "paced breathing" or "breathing pacer" computer or phone apps (many are free). Some apps even measure your breathing to help you learn the skill.

Choose what works best for you to learn and practice pacing and deepening your breathing. Don't wait until you are in crisis. A good general starting point is to breathe in for four seconds, breathe out for six seconds, pause for one second, and repeat. Then individualize from there.

Milton Z. Brown, PhD provides clear, professional paced breathing instructions, based on how it is researched to be effective, on his website, Regulating Emotions through Slow Abdominal Breathing: http://www.dbtsandiego.com/DBT2.pdf.

Progressive Muscle Relaxation

Progressive Muscle Relaxation works best when you are sitting or lying down in a comfortable position. Your eyes can be slightly open or closed, but most people find closing their eyes helps maintain focus. Loosen any tight clothing, find a quiet place, and follow these basic steps:

1. Do a minute of deep breathing before you begin.
2. Inhale slowly and deeply through your nose and exhale through your mouth. Repeat this several times.
3. Gradually work your way downward or upward, tensing then relaxing one muscle group at a time in your face, neck, shoulders, chest, arms, hands, back, stomach, buttocks, legs, and feet. Hold each tensed position for about five to ten seconds, quickly release the tension, and remain still, allowing twenty to thirty seconds of relaxation.
4. After you've completed all of the muscle groups, continue deep breathing and focus on how you feel in this relaxed state. Notice the difference between how you feel now and how you felt at the beginning of the exercise.

Quite a bit of mental focus is needed to attend to this relaxing work. It is hard to intentionally tense, count, and release specific muscle groups when your mind is somewhere else. Part of the skill is to notice when your mind wanders, which it regularly does with thoughts like, "I ate too much lunch.

This is dumb. I look so stupid. I'm doing it wrong." Then refocus your mind back onto the muscle group you're working on. As sensations like warmth and heaviness are felt in relaxed muscles after they are tensed, the sensations themselves bring a mental relaxation as well.

With practice, over time, you can learn to recognize the difference between the feeling of a tensed muscle (indicating emotional activation) and a completely relaxed muscle. Once you develop the skill, you can then choose to relax your muscles when you first notice tension. Here again, you must pay attention and notice before you can intervene. With physical relaxation comes mental calmness—in any situation. Muscle tension and mental calmness are too incompatible to coexist.

Try this: Make a tight fist and flex your hand upward at the wrist. Focus on the sensations you feel while these muscles are tensed. Hold the tensed position for about ten seconds and then completely release, relaxing your hand and arm. Let your hand and arm go limp, and let it fall. Focus on how your relaxed muscles feel. Repeat this a couple of times. Focus on the different feelings and physical sensations between tensing and relaxing your fist.

If you experience feelings of emotional distress while using PMR, stop and try another intervention. Then talk to your therapist or doctor about your difficulties. If you experience any intense muscle pain while performing this exercise, stop immediately and call your doctor.

Putting Your Worries on a Shelf is a CD on which Marsha Linehan, PhD, the developer of Dialectical Behavioral Therapy (DBT), walks the listener through the practice of progressive muscle relaxation. It was produced by Behavioral Tech, LLC (2005) and can be found on the following website in the products section:

http://behavioraltech.org/products/list.cfm?category=Compact%20Discs

Audio Instruction/CDs
Deep Breathing or Diaphragmatic Breathing
Andrew Weil, MD has instructions on his website as well as free downloads from online music sites. http://www.drweil.com/drw/u/ART00519/An-Introduction-to-Breathing.html

Breathing: The Master Key to Self Healing (The Self Healing Series) by Andrew Weil. Sounds True, Incorporated (November 1, 1999).

Additional Resources

Websites
The following are websites with vast resources. They are well-known and respected sources of information and help for individuals with eating disorders, their loved ones, caring others, professionals, and the general public.

National Eating Disorders Association (NEDA)
http://www.nationaleatingdisorders.org/information-resources/general-information.php#body-image-issues

Proud 2B Me is a website created by NEDA for teens who struggle with eating disorders and related issues.
http://proud2bme.org/

National Association of Anorexia Nervosa and Associated Disorders (ANAD)
http://www.anad.org/get-information/about-eating-disorders/eating-disorders-statistics/

Eating Disorders Resources for Recovery is a website is provided by Gurze Books, Inc., which is a great place to find the full range of books about eating disorders. They publish a web newsletter and provide information about education, events, organizations, and referrals, all of which are found on this site.
http://www.bulimia.com

Books

Intuitive Eating: A Revolutionary Program That Works, Evelyn Tribole and Elyse Resch. Third Edition, 2012, St. Martin's Griffin.

Life without Ed, Jenni Schaefer and Thom Rutledge. 2003, McGraw-Hill.

Goodbye Ed, Hello Me, Jenni Schaefer. 2009, McGraw-Hill.

End Emotional Eating: Using Dialectical Behavior Therapy Skills to Cope with Difficult Emotions and Develop a Healthy Relationship to Food, Jennifer L. Taitz, PsyD. 2012, New Harbinger Publications, Inc.

Unofficial Guide to Managing Eating Disorders, Sara Dulaney Gilbert. 2000, Wiley Publishing, Inc.

Help Your Teenager Beat an Eating Disorder, James Lock and Daniel Le Grange. 2005, Guilford Press.

Feel the Fear . . . and Do It Anyway, Susan Jeffers, PhD. 1987, Ballantine Books.

Support
Eating Disorders Anonymous
http://www.eatingdisordersanonymous.org/

Alcoholics Anonymous
http://www.aa.org/